Nancy Herman

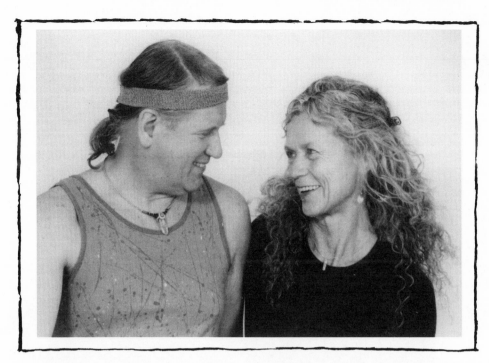

ISBN number: 0-9664255-2-9

Library of Congress Catalog Card Number:
2003108265

GANESHA PRESS   First Edition

1563 Solano Avenue, Box 144
Berkeley, CA 94707. U.S.A.
web address: www.angela-victor.com

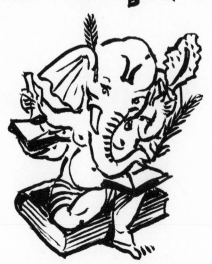

From Inside Out

BOOK THREE

A YOGA NOTE BOOK from the teachings of
ANGELA and VICTOR

by

Victor van Kooten

BODY ENERGY

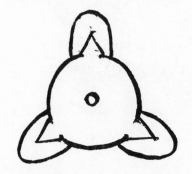

for more information about the workshops:
www. angela – victor. com

o hand written text and art-work
by : Victor van Kooten
with the exception of the 2 pages
by: David King and Robert Paschell.

I would like to thank Ellen Toomey for all
her love, time and energy poured into the
birth and distribution of the two previous
books "From Inside Out" and now Book III,
"Body Energy".
I also would like to thank
David King for proof-reading all the material.

To Me
Every page is a kōan
as Every pose is a kōan .
Giving your full attention,
a sudden breeze might move
the heavy curtain
for a split second
exposing Sa-lo-me,
fa-re-do, dancing:
the naked truth
of your mind.

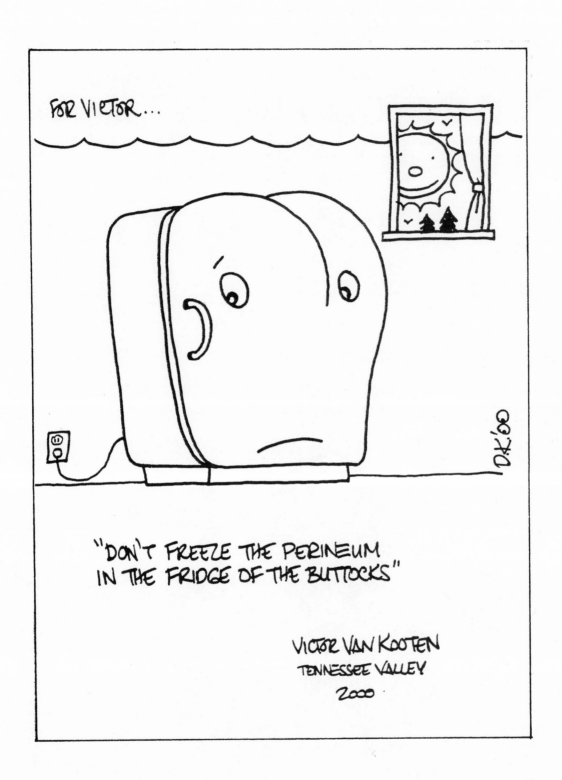

Thanks to David King.

the human form,
the function,
is there
a
Clue?

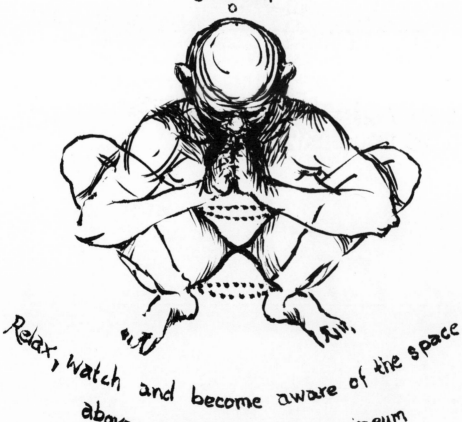

for me yoga is
a way to
study the magnificence
of
creation
o

Relax, watch and become aware of the space
above, underneath the perineum
and let the energy
flow...

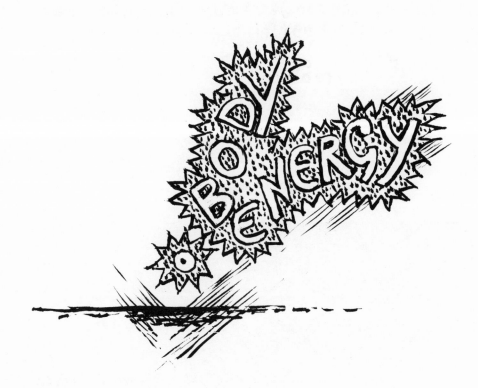

You can put a potato in a bag, put the bag in a cupboard, put the cupboard in a room, come back a month later, go into the room, open the cupboard, open the bag, and there will be the pale arms of the potato, reaching for its lost lover, the sun. A seed in the ground knows where the sun is. Knows which way to reach for fire or water, and lives somewhere in between. You can separate yourself from yourself, from nature, from God, from the communion and suffering of others, but inside you is a light seeking release from your body's darkness, and an invisible seed reaching for the light. The flow of currents there is what we call life.

Shadows are very seductive, very mysterious. I wonder what lies down that dark alleyway, hmmm…? The ten thousand things are robed in a shimmering cloak of nuance. Break the mold of definition to find the light. How? One way is to sit quietly like a potato till your blind eyes sprout leaf-fringed arms.

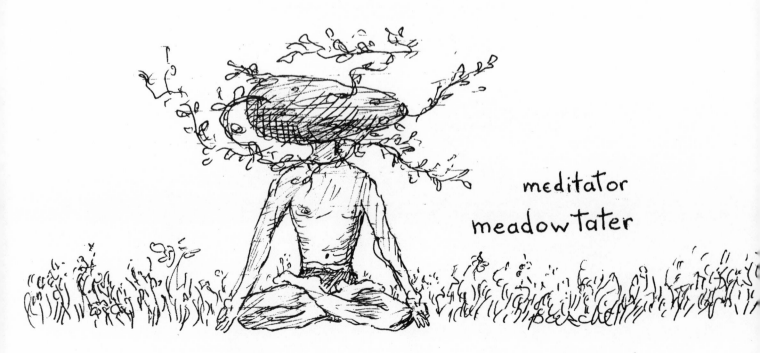

meditator
meadow tater

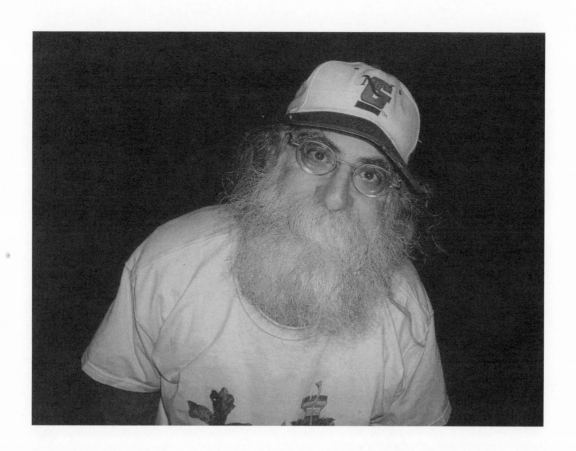

Robert Paschell walks in the woods, creates things, and goofs off in Yellow Springs, Ohio. Check out his artwork on T-shirts at www.improbablebob.netfirms.com, or send him a potato recipe at rpaschell@yahoo.com. And remember: To make an ॐ "OM"-let you've got to break some egos!

We met Robert some 10 years ago during a Jazz - Session, where he was reading his poetry. Whenever we teach in Yellow Springs, we often bump into each other, as we wonder around town.

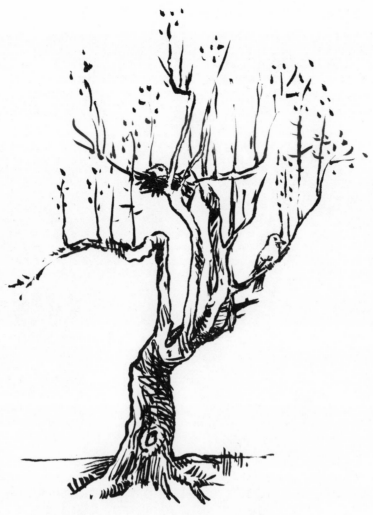

Knowledge can never replace
          the real thing.
We know a tree will grow from
a single tiny seed, with all the
potential of hosting bugs and birds.

  But only when it has actually grown
into a mature fruit-bearing tree,
can we tell if it is a wood pigeon

      or a wood pecker.

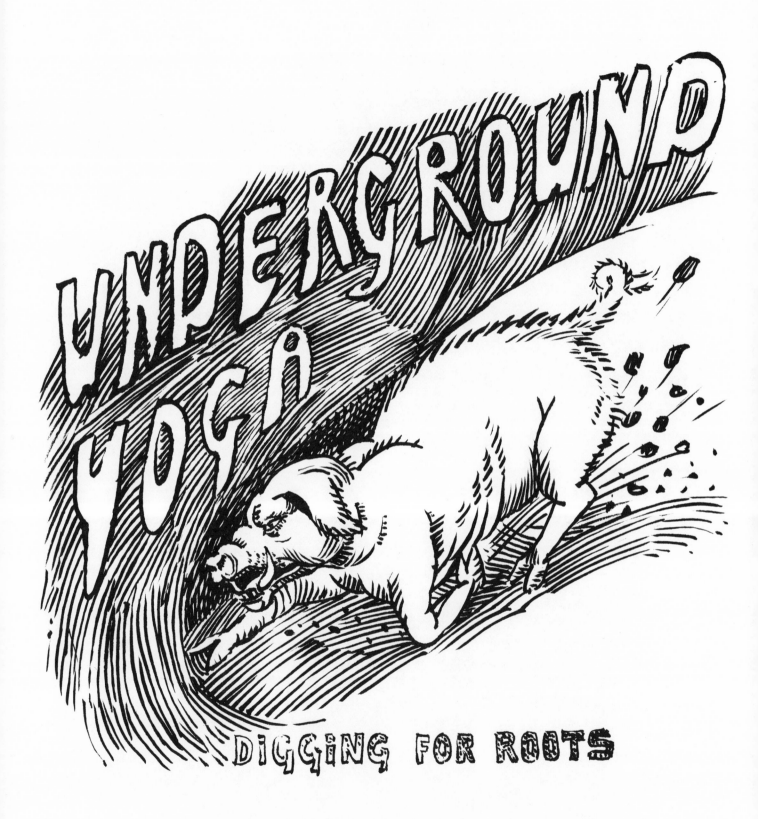

A story that describes the energy which underlies all of Creation: Is there a beginning and end to Shiva's Lingam? When this question was put before Vishnu, he incarnated into a wild boar and dug deep down into the Earth, only to return to Shiva admitting that he was unable to find any beginning. When Brahma was asked this question, he mounted his Swan and circled higher and higher, but unsuccessful to find the end of the Lingam. Unwilling to admit to failure, he asked a falling blossom to help him in convincing Shiva they both had found the end. Shiva tells them this is an absolute lie. For this Brahma will never have his own temple for worship and the blossom can never be used in any sacred ritual ....

From one single unified truth, the
ever changing reality of our world,
where truth and lie go hand in hand.
Pointing to the transformation from
this duality into the infinite
power of the the Life force itself,
which will happen when your Vishnu
and Brahma search for the limits of who
you are.

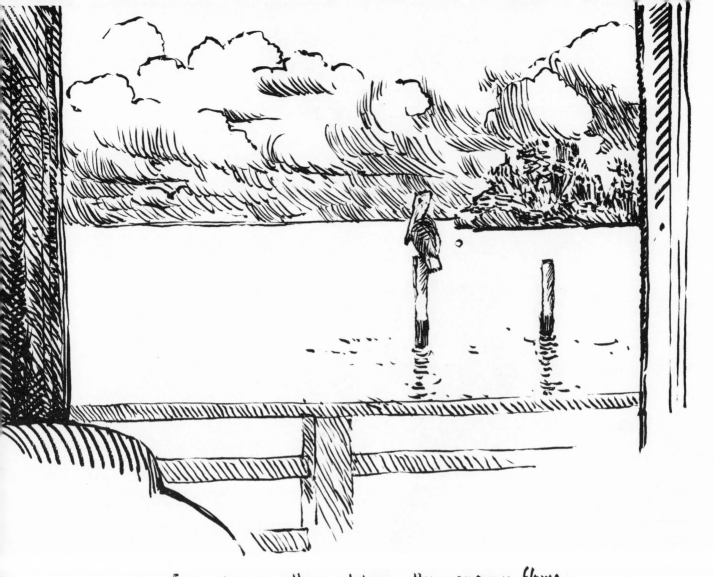

first space, then vision. Now energy flows
and our body moves.
drawn out off a silent state
we come
to
movement

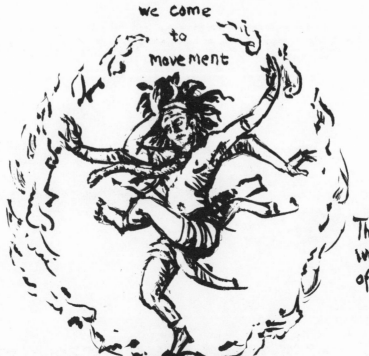

Through Shiva's dance
we become aware
of the silent center.

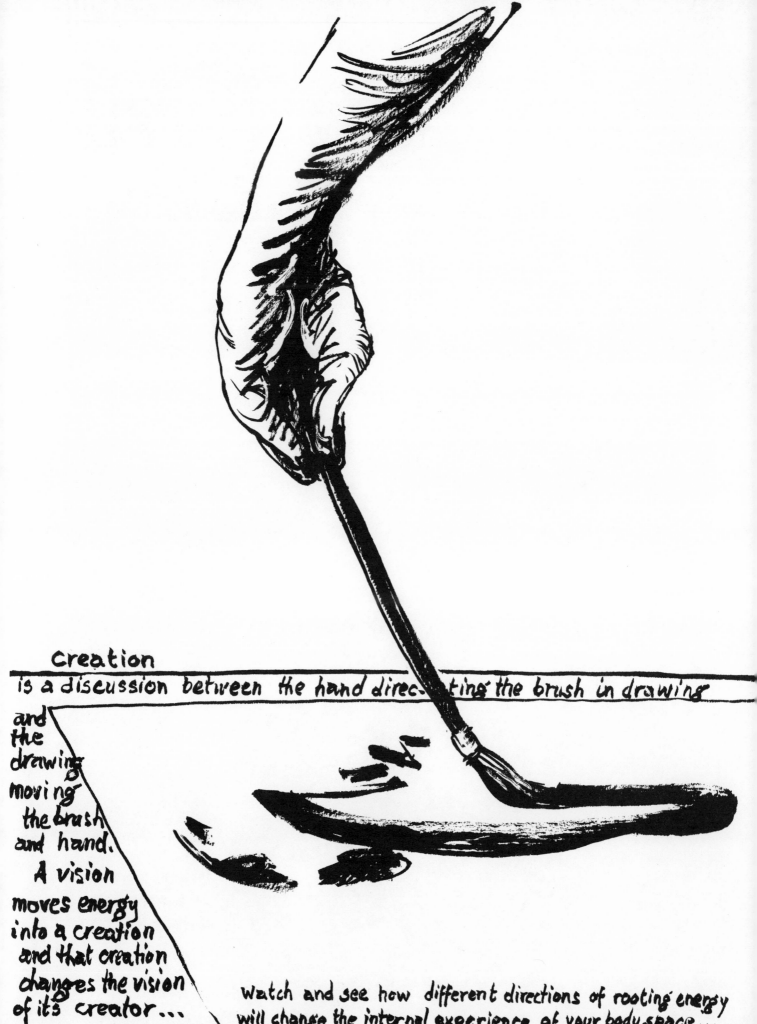

Creation
is a discussion between the hand direc-ting the brush in drawing
and
the
drawing
moving
the brush
and hand.
A vision
moves energy
into a creation
and that creation
changes the vision
of its creator...

Watch and see how different directions of rooting energy
will change the internal experience of your body space...

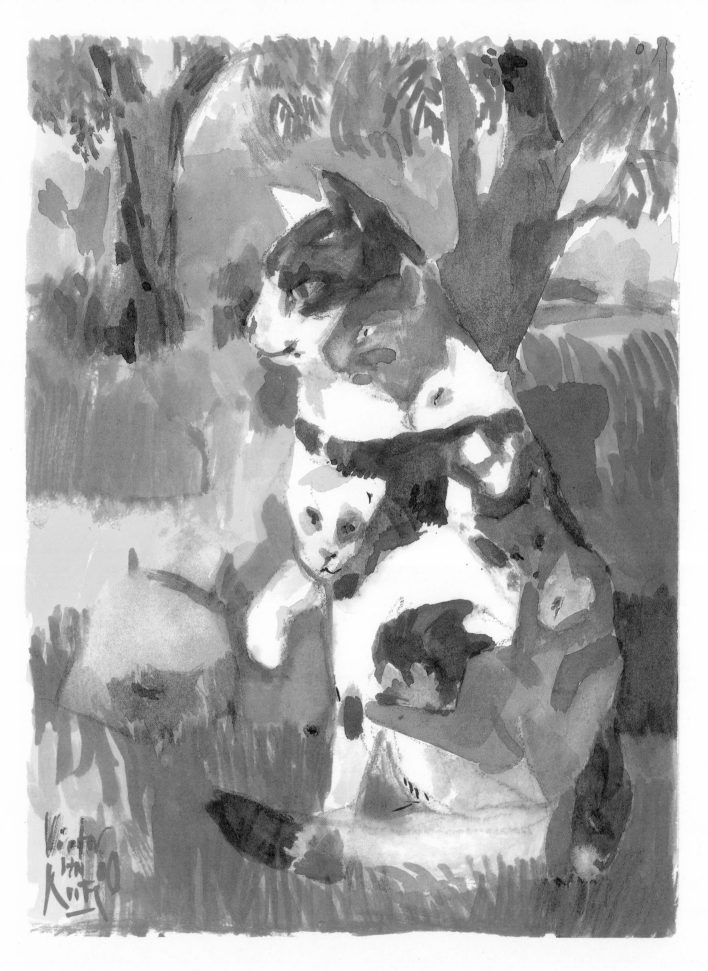

don't even ask me who my parents were...

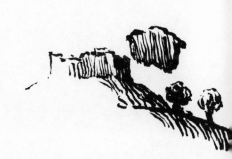

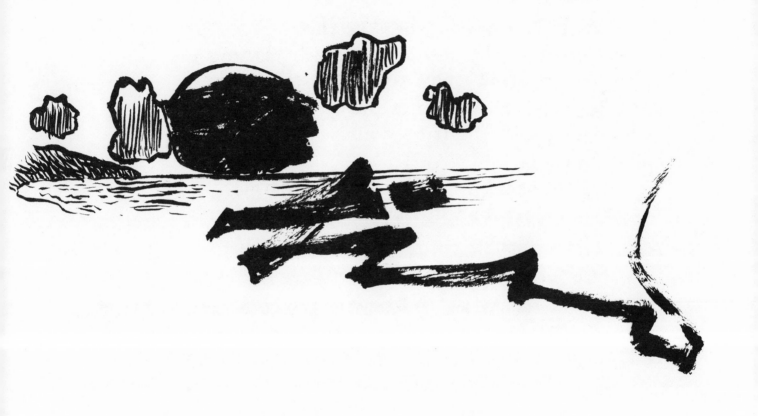

The White Pure Energy gets stained...
   awareness starts to choose direction
      towards itself

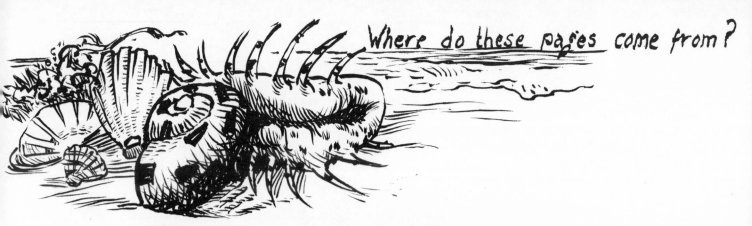

When you walk the beach
and pick up the shells that catch your eye,
do you realise they are not numbered?
    They are thrown onto the beach after
the slugs and shellfish died.
        Likewise
            the pages of my books are forms
                left behind by my thoughts.

    If you pick up their shape and words,
    you will decide upon their page number.

        As for me, I honestly try to accept all thoughts
            and especially those that make no sense.
    By allowing the black ink to flow, I witness the
    complexity of human existence.
            I will see the double meanings,
            the HA and THA of it all,

            the right and left hand of God
                    Creating
            Not only "in the beginning"
                but constantly Now...

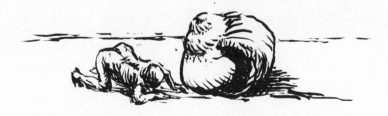

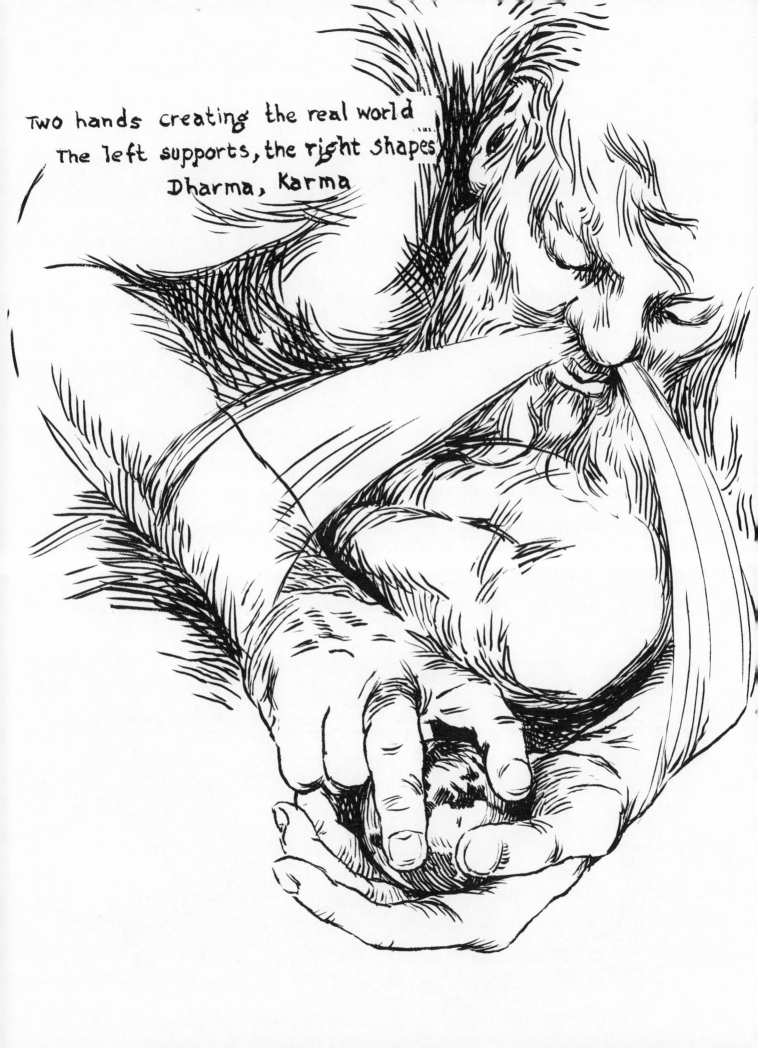

Two hands creating the real world
The left supports, the right shapes
Dharma, Karma

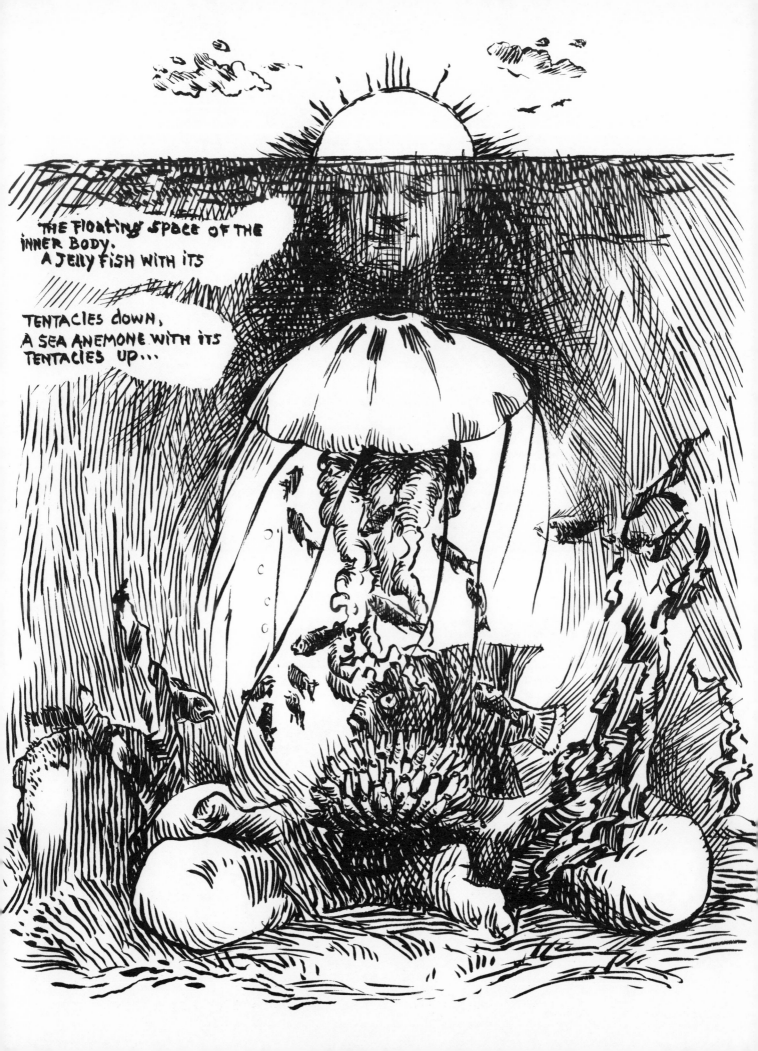

SUSUMNA

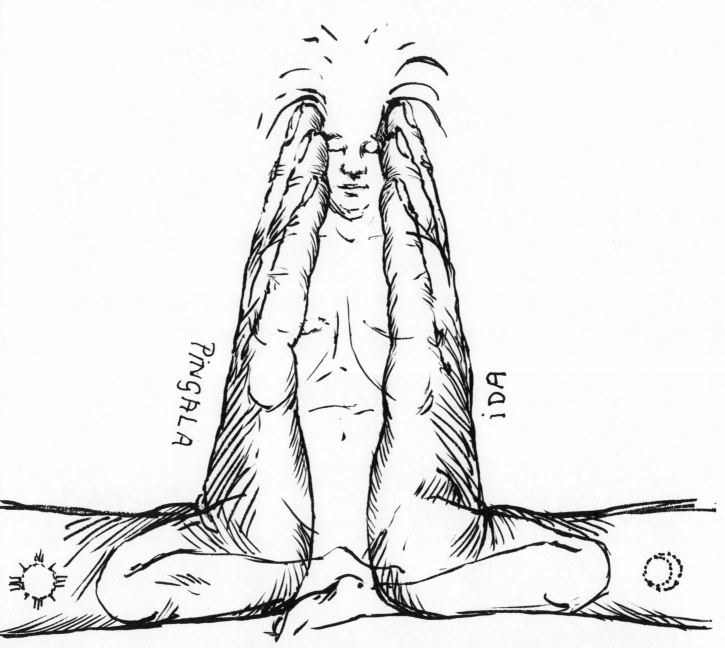

PINGALA

IDA

In Yoga asana we pray with the physical in order to connect
with the great, invisible Source, making use of duality
to come to and into Unity. All effects, flexibility, health, etc.,
   sprouting from this practise, are trivial and not the reason
for this practise. Yoga asana is a prayer that brings creation
back home where it belongs: in the hands of the Creator.

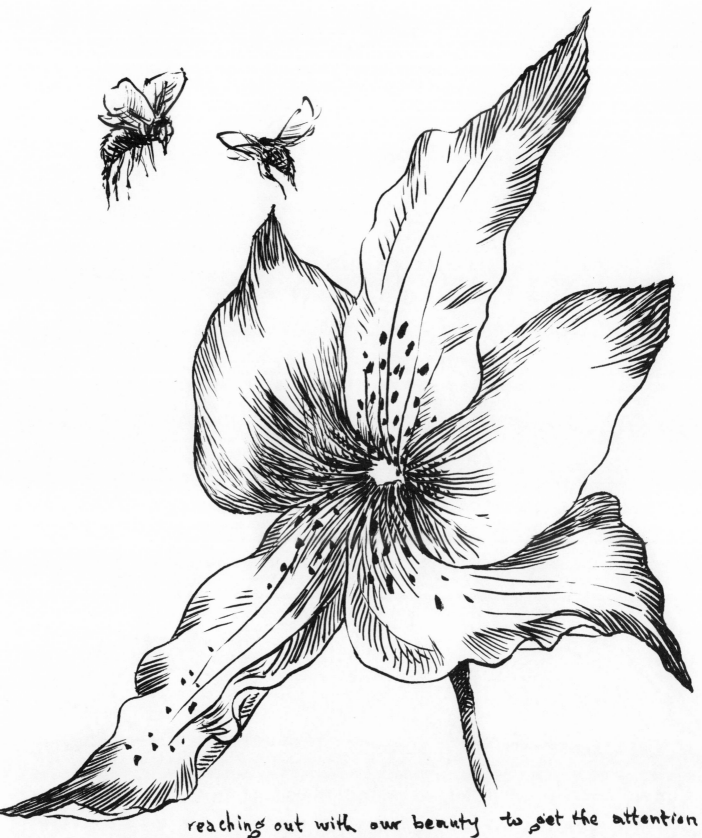

reaching out with our beauty to get the attention
flying towards our empty center...

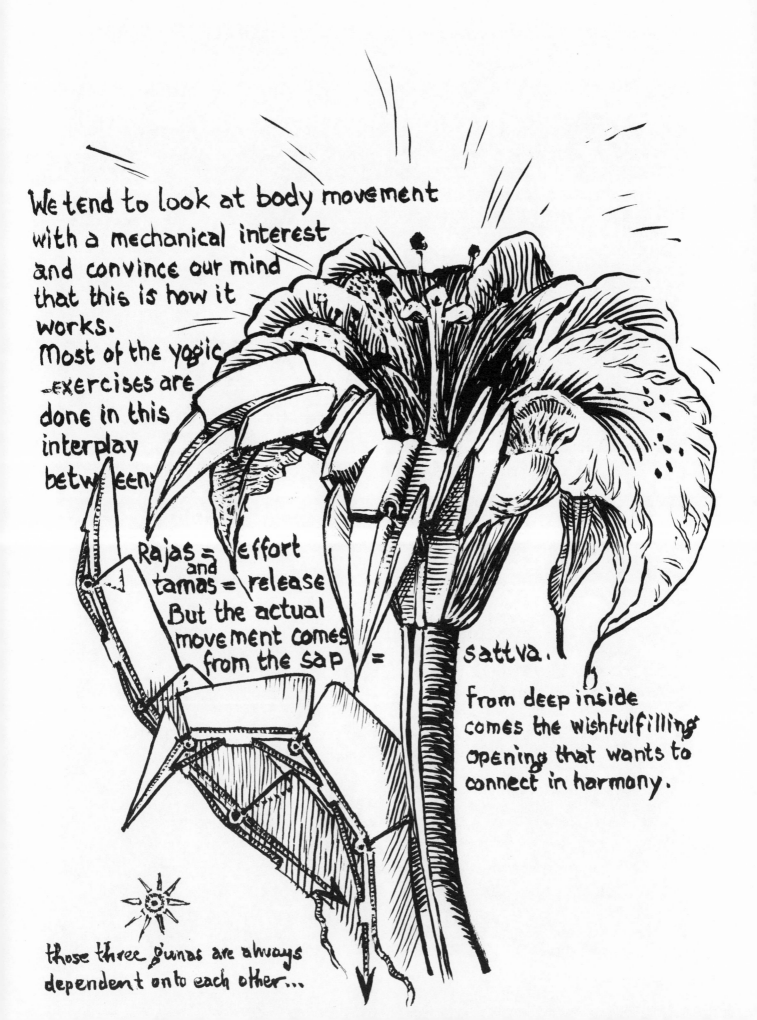

We tend to look at body movement
with a mechanical interest
and convince our mind
that this is how it
works.
Most of the yogic
exercises are
done in this
interplay
between:

Rajas = effort
and
tamas = release
But the actual
movement comes
from the sap = sattva.

From deep inside
comes the wishfulfilling
opening that wants to
connect in harmony.

those three gunas are always
dependent onto each other...

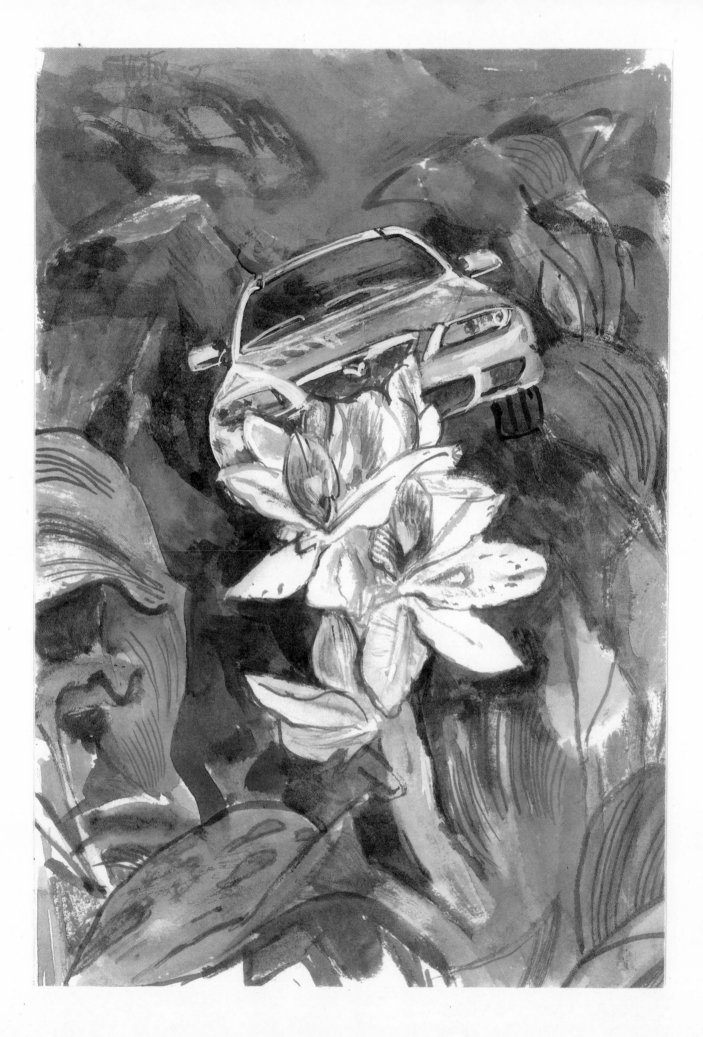

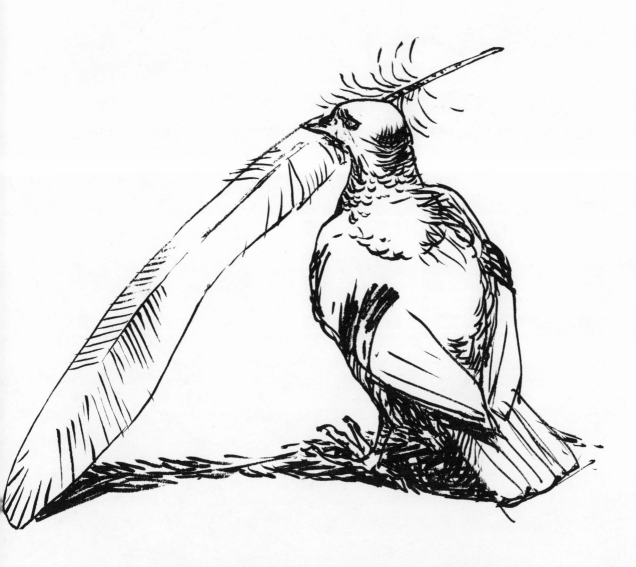

some one else's feathers will slow you down.

Fascination with some one else's support system (dharma)
takes you out of your own life.

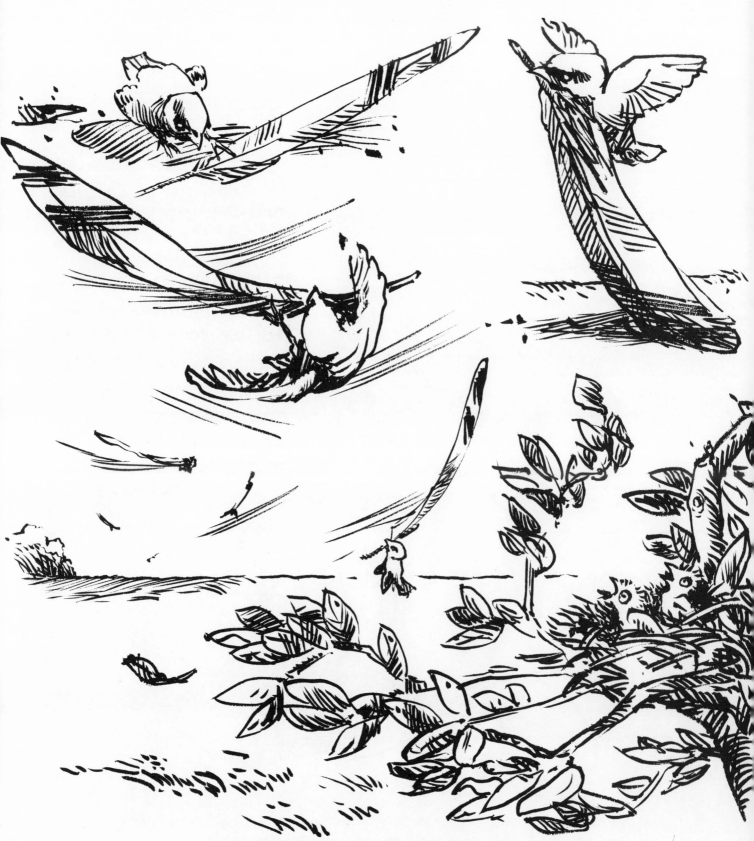

all they saw, was a fast disappearing dot over the horizon...

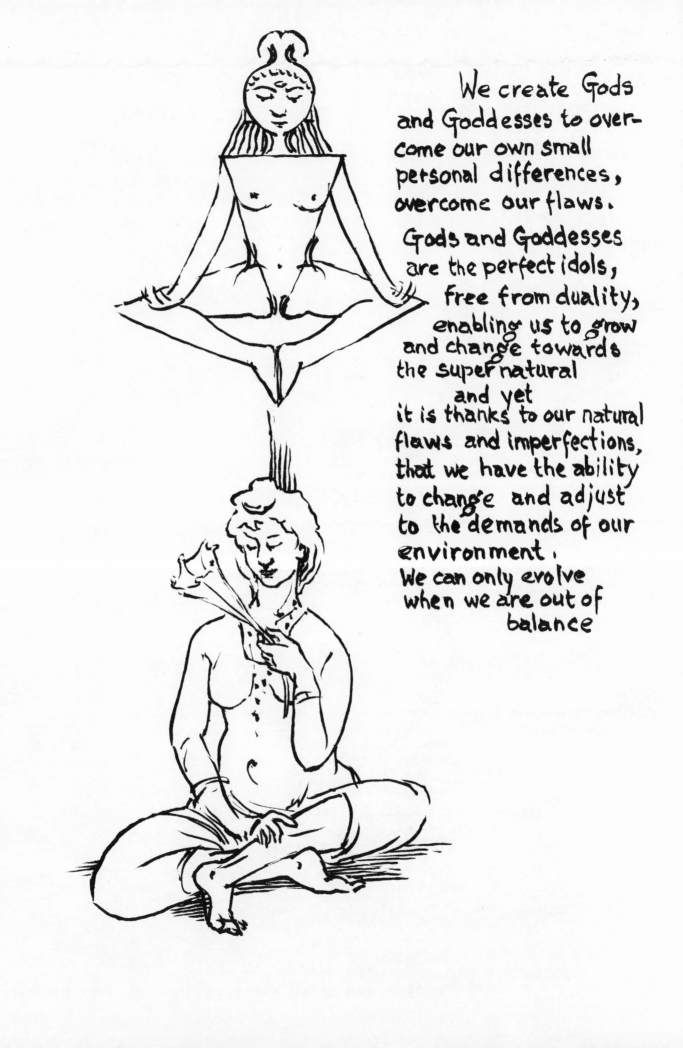

We create Gods
and Goddesses to over-
come our own small
personal differences,
overcome our flaws.

Gods and Goddesses
are the perfect idols,
   free from duality,
   enabling us to grow
and change towards
the supernatural
      and yet
it is thanks to our natural
flaws and imperfections,
that we have the ability
to change and adjust
to the demands of our
environment.
We can only evolve
when we are out of
      balance

GOD
The Masks of the Creator

Everything a part of Creation also has the great full and it may Become without your given

that becomes the endless and has form a link to formless, solid as appear, aware destroying own world.

out of its own
needless need
making its own
invisible form
visible.

detachment happens when you fully embrace
the world.

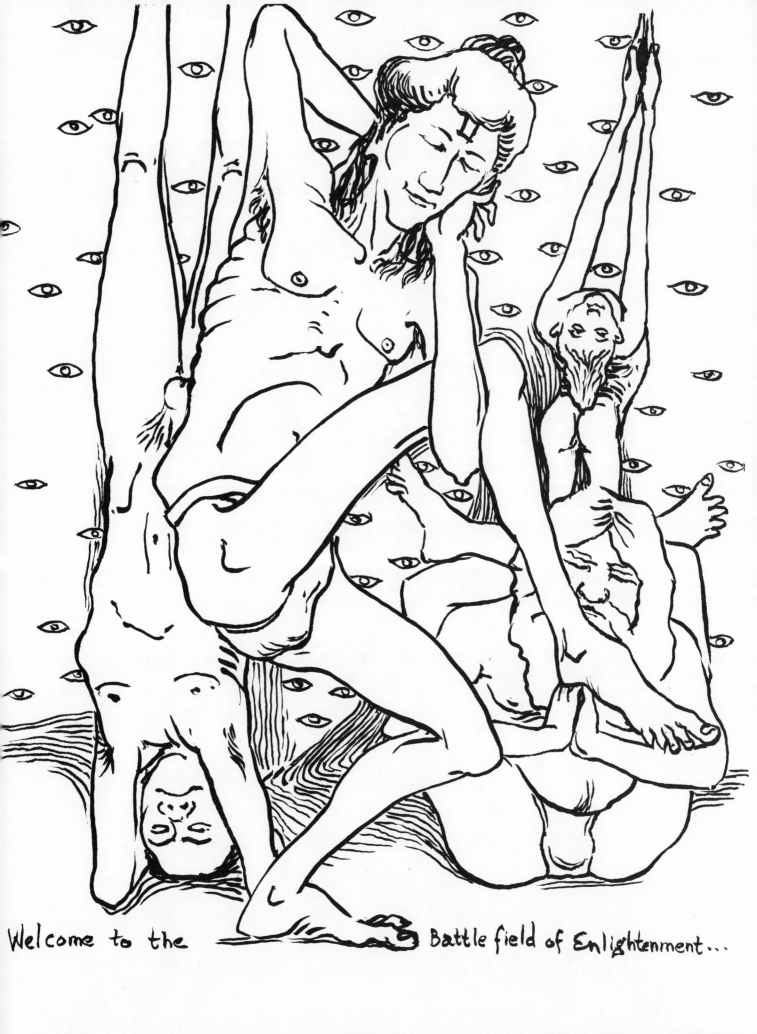

Welcome to the ————— Battle field of Enlightenment...

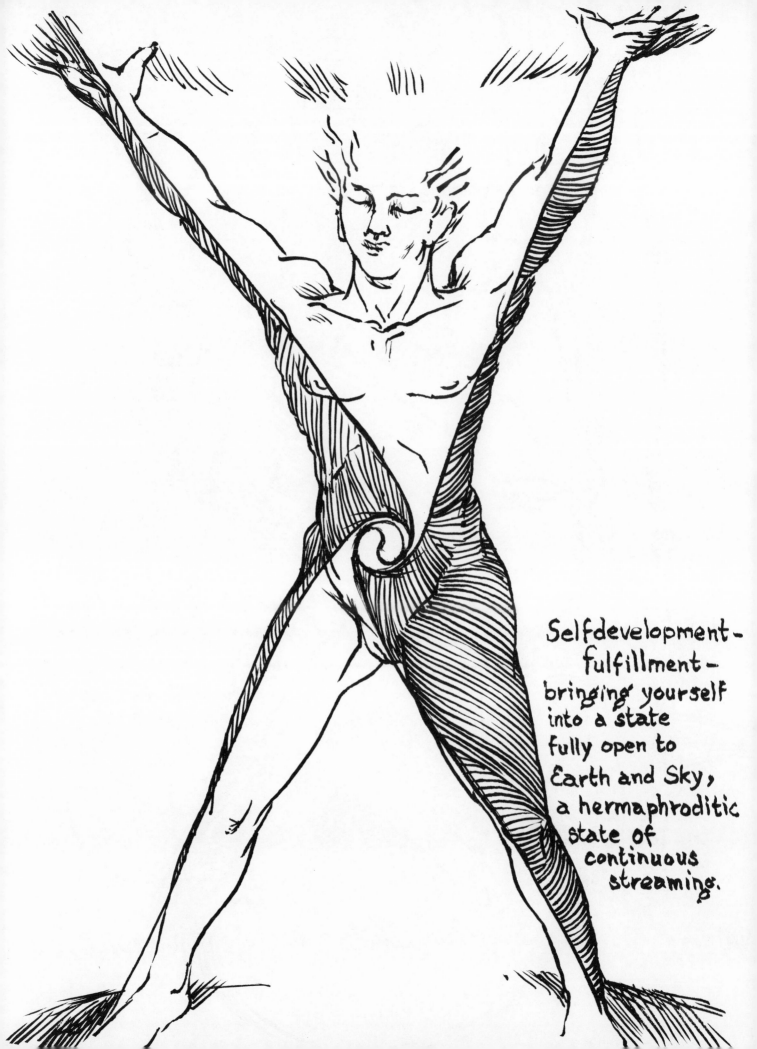

Selfdevelopment -
fulfillment -
bringing yourself
into a state
fully open to
Earth and Sky,
a hermaphroditic
state of
continuous
streaming.

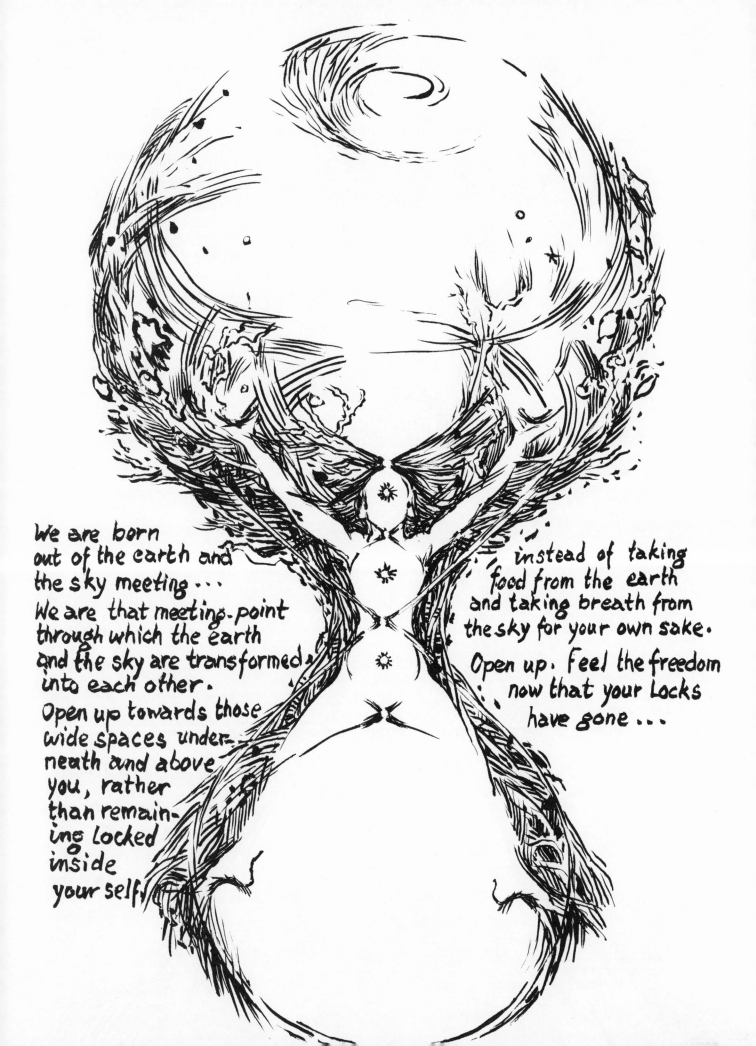

We are born
out of the earth and
the sky meeting...
We are that meeting-point
through which the earth
and the sky are transformed
into each other.
Open up towards those
wide spaces under-
neath and above
you, rather
than remain-
ing locked
inside
your self,

instead of taking
food from the earth
and taking breath from
the sky for your own sake.

Open up. Feel the freedom
now that your locks
have gone...

Three Stages of the exhalation
The birth of the
Cosmic Egg

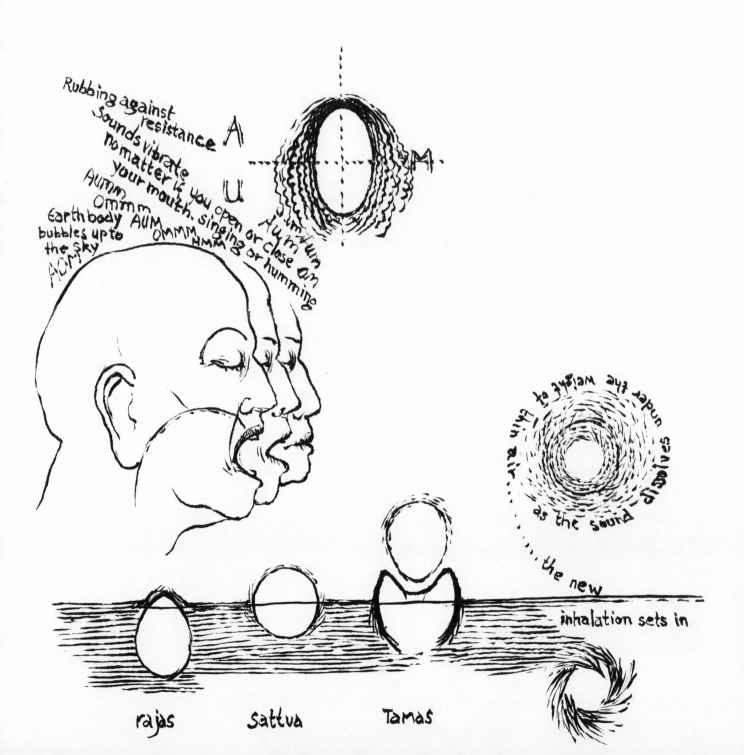

Rubbing against resistance

A U M

Sounds vibrate no matter if you open or close your mouth, singing or humming

Aumm
Ommm
Earth body AUM
bubbles up to OMMM HMM
the sky AUMM

Aum/um

under the weight of their own dissolves
as the sound dissolves

.... the new

inhalation sets in

rajas   sattva   Tamas

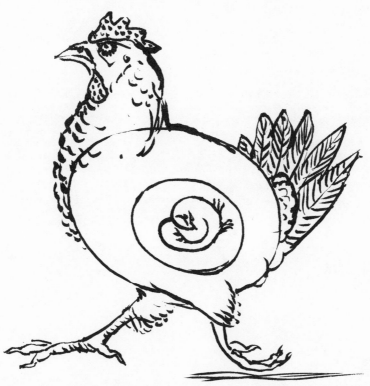

About the question of "who came first: the chicken or the egg?", there is not much to say, since they are both one. The egg is a more condensed form and it is all a matter of interest. If you are into consuming chicken, you will pat the egg first, otherwise there will be no chicken waiting for you. If you only eat eggs, your interest will be in the chicken who will have to lay them for you, which makes the chicken number one for you. If you are vegetarian you can be more detached and see them both as one: Walking eggs is chicken, dreaming chicken is egg.

About form: Can we believe what we see?

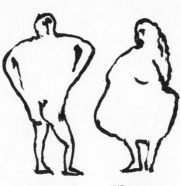

man   woman.

What is creating shapes?
Is energy creating a specific form or are forms just accidental and to be completely ignored?

opening to heaven

opening to Earth

receiving their forces, funneling and compressing them.

life continues when man meets woman and they lose themselves in each other.

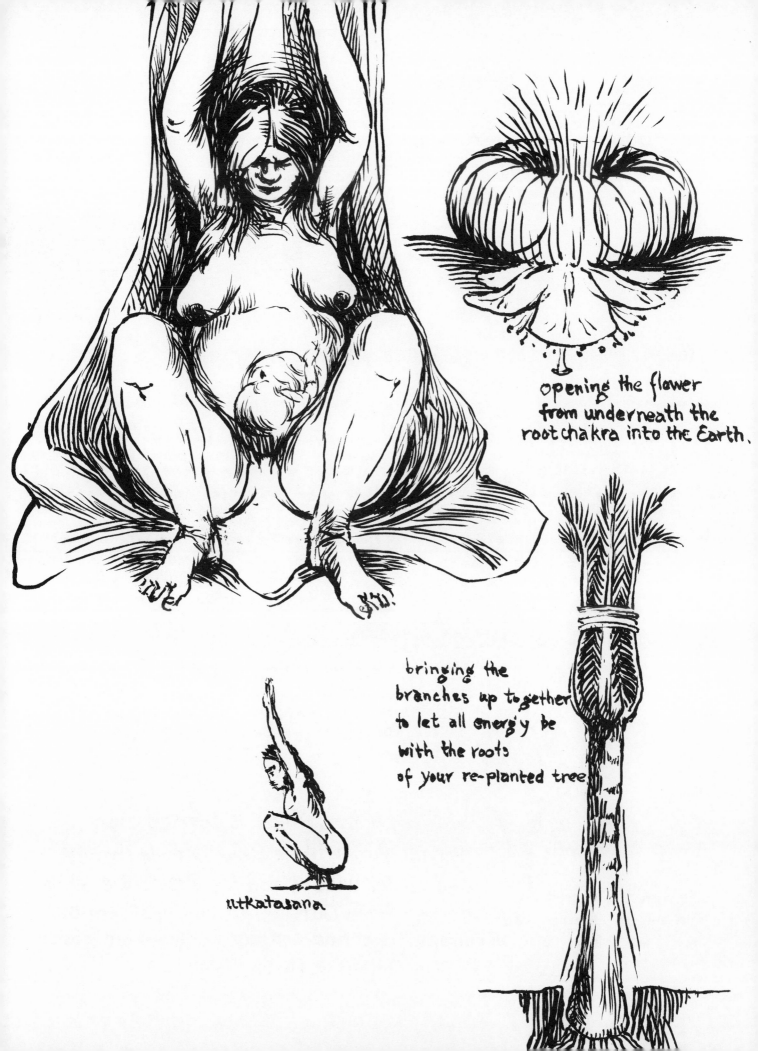

opening the flower
from underneath the
root chakra into the Earth.

bringing the
branches up together
to let all energy be
with the roots
of your re-planted tree

utkatasana

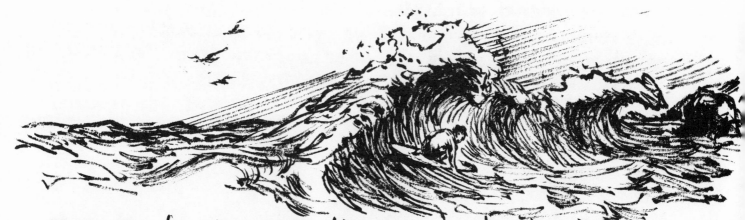

The surfer has to await the wave and ride...
We simply have no power over the ocean
no matter how far we swim out.

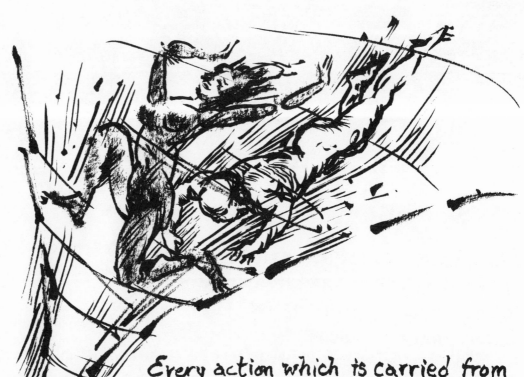

Every action which is carried from
Inside Out, will be clear, simple, honest
and easily understood by everyone, while
moving from Outside in will be strenuous,
full of effort and confuses communication.

words of   a falling angel, a failing angel.

Transformation.

The stages in life become symbolic statements that nothing remains the same. Through letting go of one form, we move towards a renewal which allows us to continue on to the next level. In the yogic state we come to realise the multiple meanings of all these layers at once, freed from the protection of the walls that keep seasons apart.

And since we live in time
and space, we live from
one moment into
the next, rather
than "in the moment",
the only moment
possible.

Each
moment
has its
own reality.

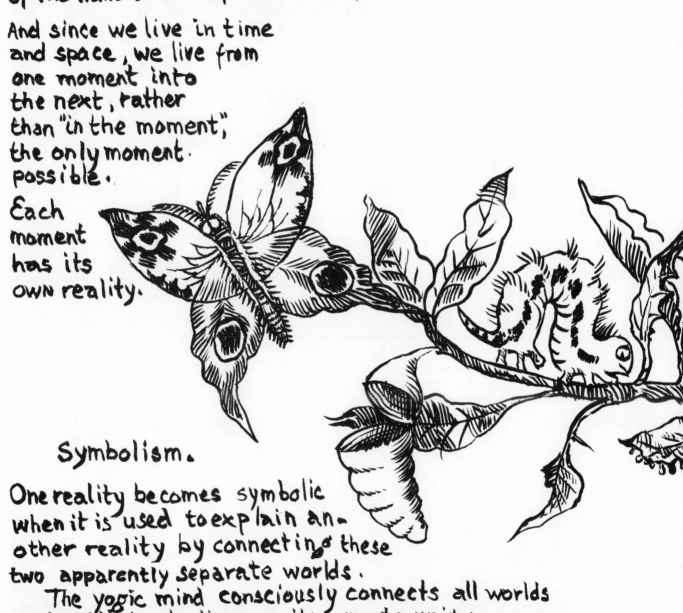

Symbolism.

One reality becomes symbolic when it is used to explain another reality by connecting these two apparently separate worlds.

The yogic mind consciously connects all worlds and melts borderlines on its way to unity.

It is only there that we realise we can not kill without killing a part of ourselves. We can not ignore anyone or anything without ignoring a part of ourselves.

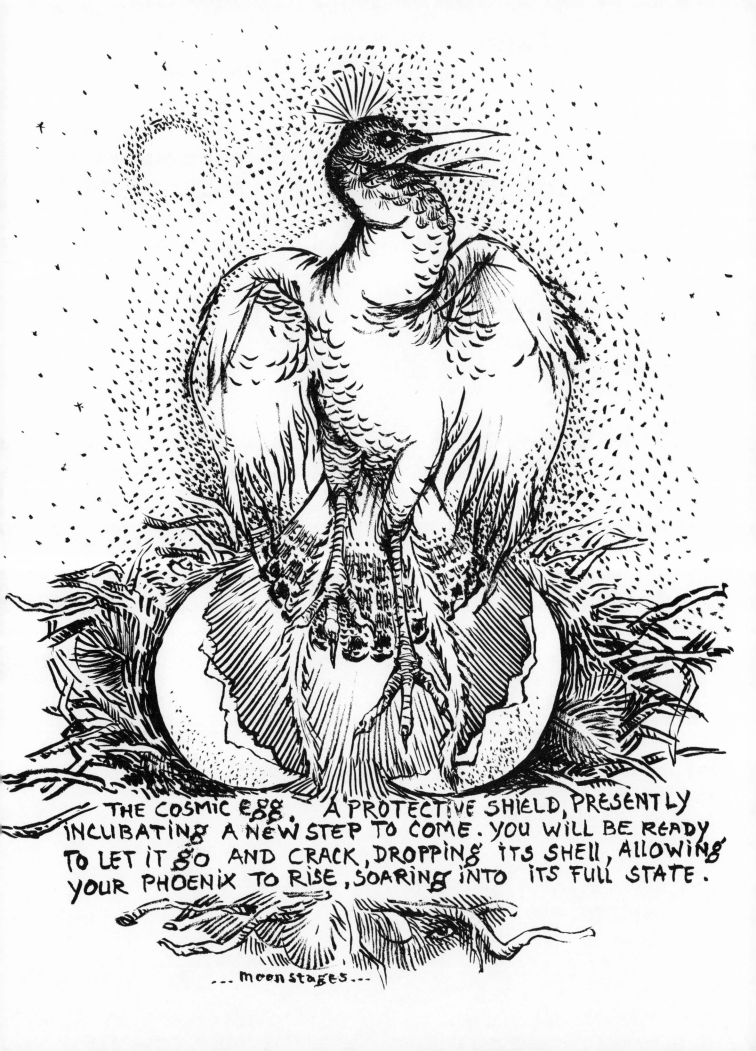

THE COSMIC egg. A PROTECTIVE SHIELD, PRESENTLY INCUBATING A NEW STEP TO COME. YOU WILL BE READY TO LET IT gO AND CRACK, DROPPING ITS SHELL, ALLOWING YOUR PHOENIX TO RISE, SOARING INTO ITS FULL STATE.

...moon stages...

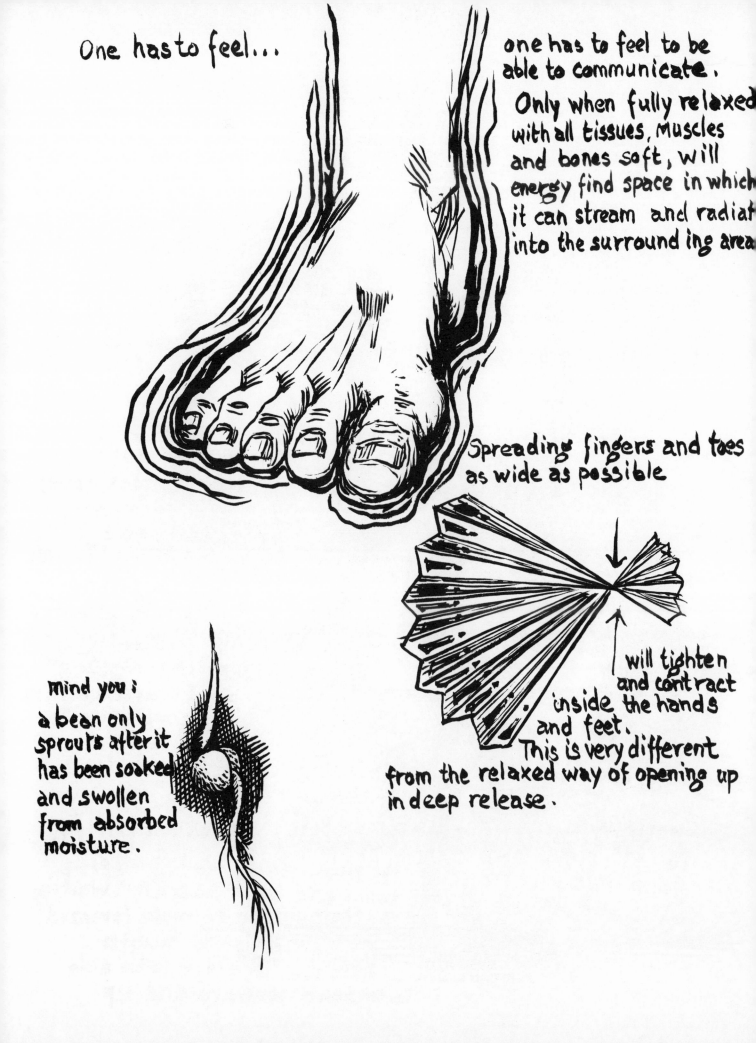

One has to feel...

one has to feel to be able to communicate.
Only when fully relaxed with all tissues, muscles and bones soft, will energy find space in which it can stream and radiate into the surrounding area.

Spreading fingers and toes as wide as possible

will tighten and contract inside the hands and feet.
This is very different from the relaxed way of opening up in deep release.

mind you:
a bean only sprouts after it has been soaked and swollen from absorbed moisture.

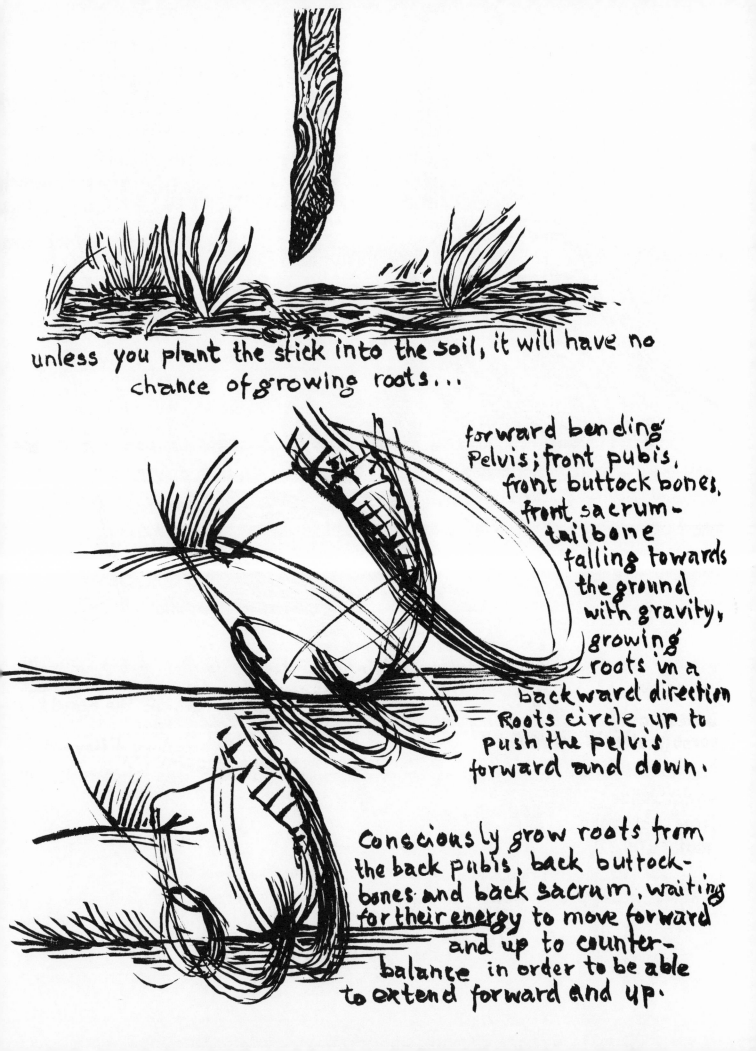

unless you plant the stick into the soil, it will have no chance of growing roots...

forward bending Pelvis; front pubis, front buttock bones, front sacrum - tailbone falling towards the ground with gravity, growing roots in a backward direction. Roots circle up to push the pelvis forward and down.

Consciously grow roots from the back pubis, back buttock-bones and back sacrum, waiting for their energy to move forward and up to counter-balance in order to be able to extend forward and up.

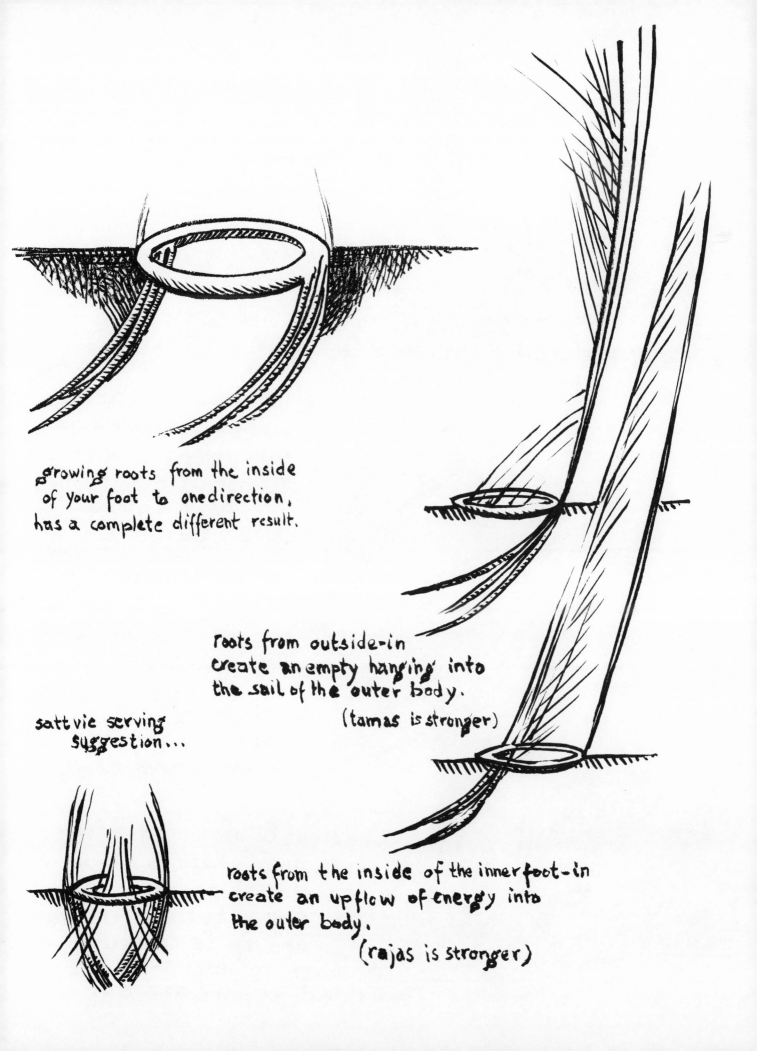

growing roots from the inside
of your foot to one direction,
has a complete different result.

roots from outside-in
create an empty hanging into
the sail of the outer body.
(tamas is stronger)

sattvic serving
suggestion...

roots from the inside of the inner foot-in
create an upflow of energy into
the outer body.
(rajas is stronger)

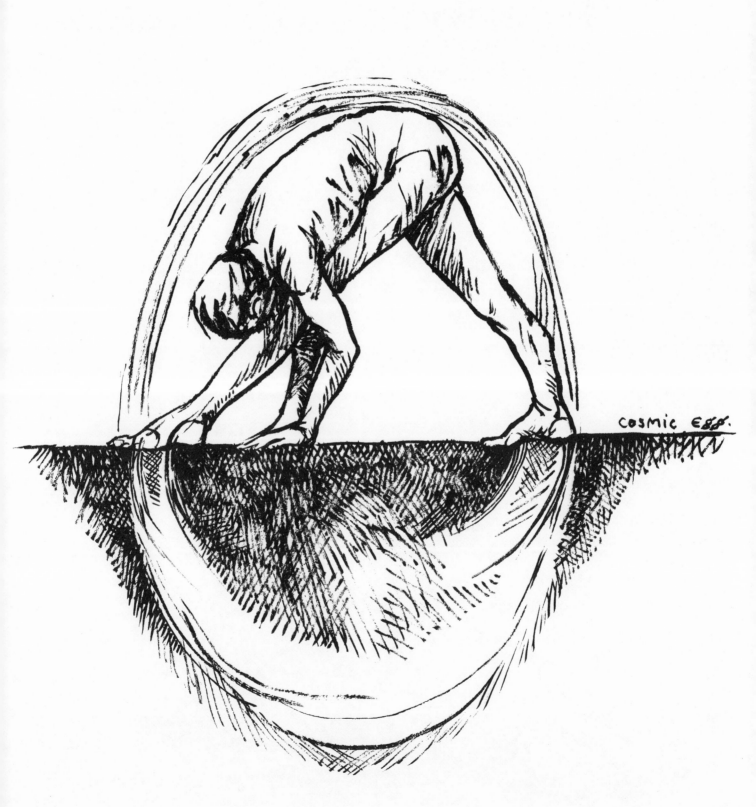

COSMIC EGG.

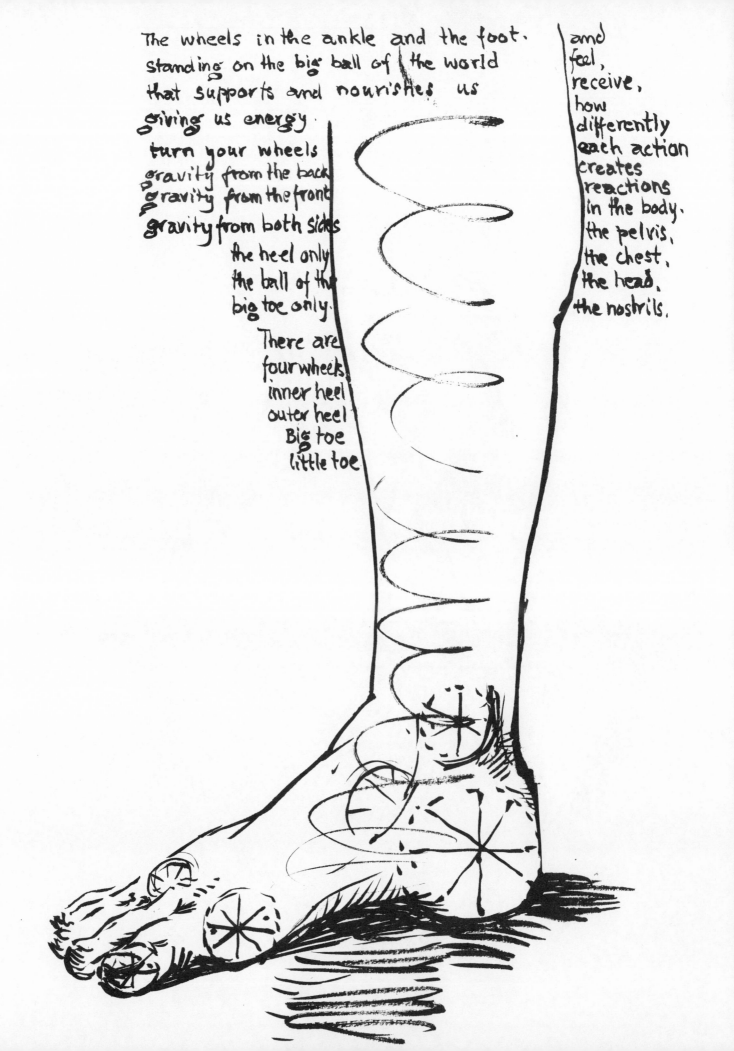

The wheels in the ankle and the foot.
standing on the big ball of the world
that supports and nourishes us
giving us energy.

turn your wheels
gravity from the back
gravity from the front
gravity from both sides

the heel only
the ball of the
big toe only.

There are
four wheels
inner heel
outer heel
Big toe
little toe

and
feel,
receive,
how
differently
each action
creates
reactions
in the body.
the pelvis,
the chest,
the head,
the nostrils.

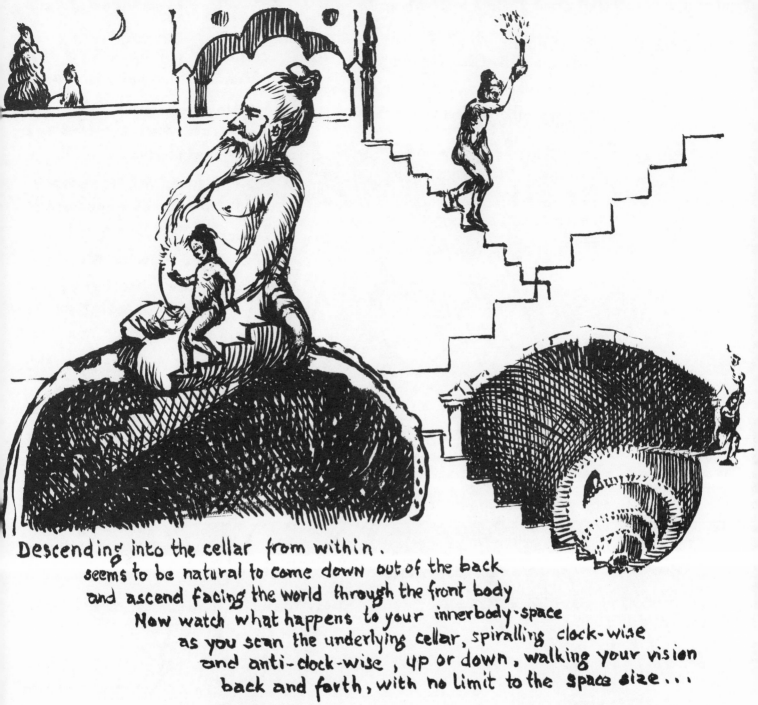

Descending into the cellar from within.
 seems to be natural to come down out of the back
 and ascend facing the world through the front body
  Now watch what happens to your innerbody-space
    as you scan the underlying cellar, spiralling clock-wise
      and anti-clock-wise, up or down, walking your vision
        back and forth, with no limit to the space size...

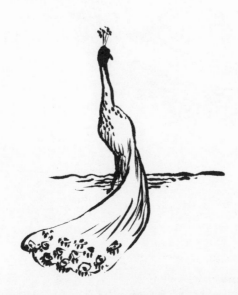

The rabbit in the moon

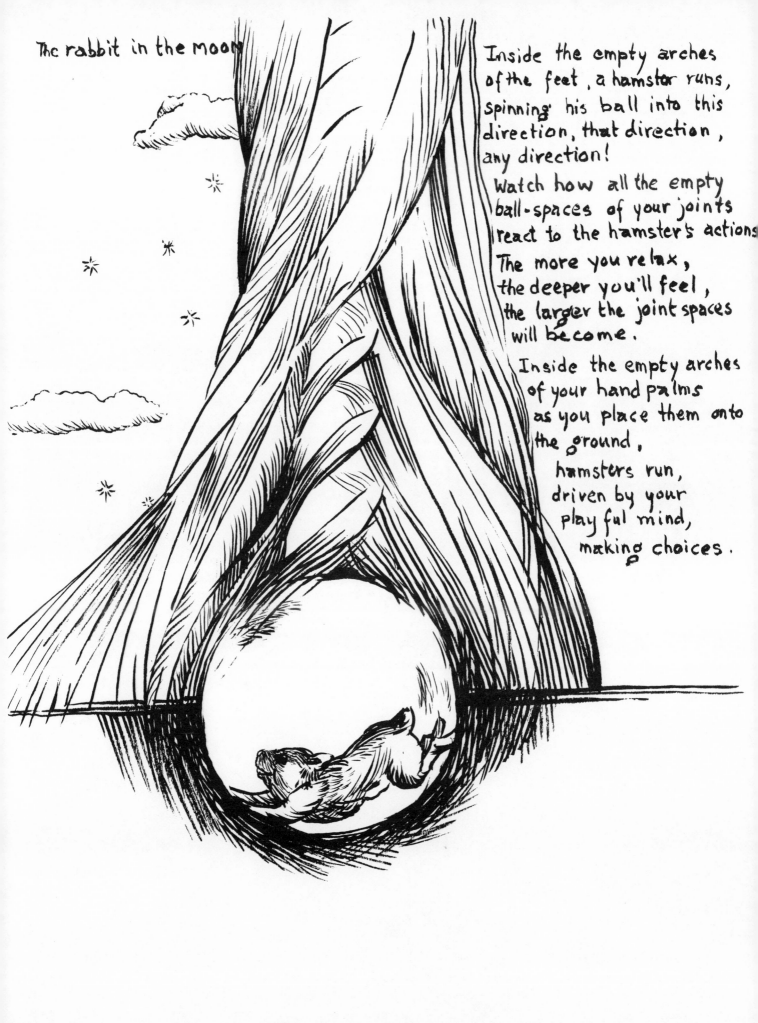

Inside the empty arches
of the feet, a hamster runs,
spinning his ball into this
direction, that direction,
any direction!
Watch how all the empty
ball-spaces of your joints
react to the hamster's actions.
The more you relax,
the deeper you'll feel,
the larger the joint spaces
will become.
Inside the empty arches
of your hand palms
as you place them onto
the ground,
hamsters run,
driven by your
playful mind,
making choices.

Standing on the wine cellar of the Gods.

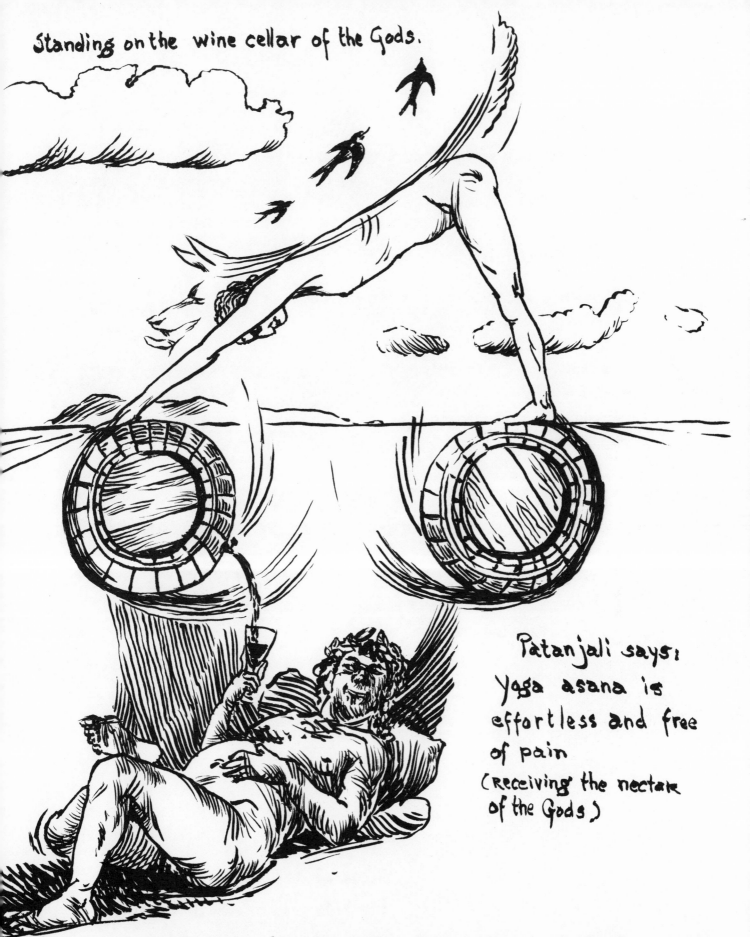

Patanjali says:
yoga asana is
effortless and free
of pain
(receiving the nectar
of the Gods)

Let the earth turn like two barrels underneath your hands and feet
and drink the energy you will receive.

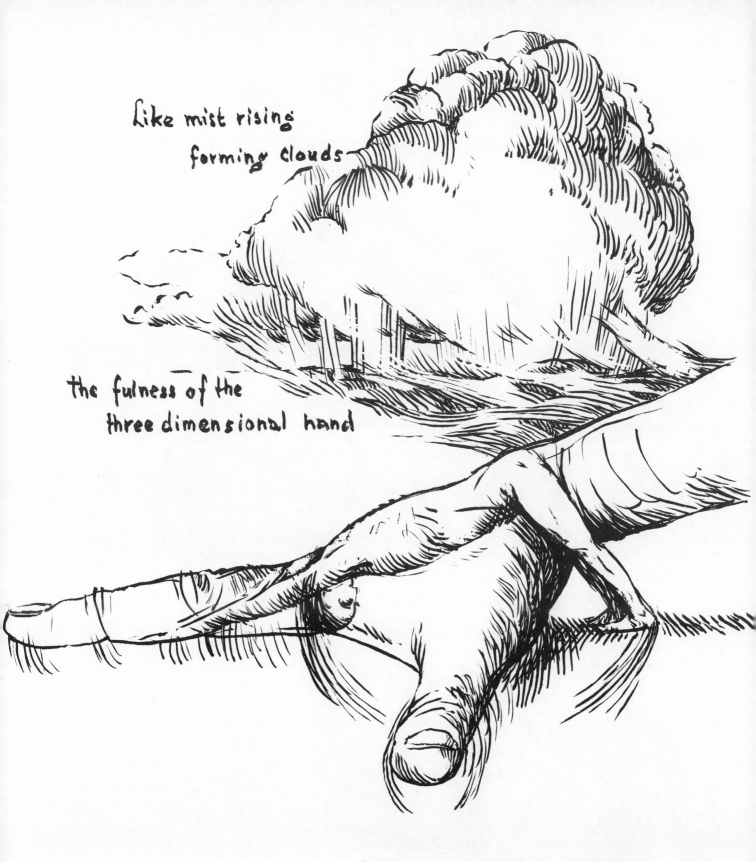

Like mist rising
forming clouds

the fulness of the
three dimensional hand

becomes the fulness of the
whole body in down-dog.

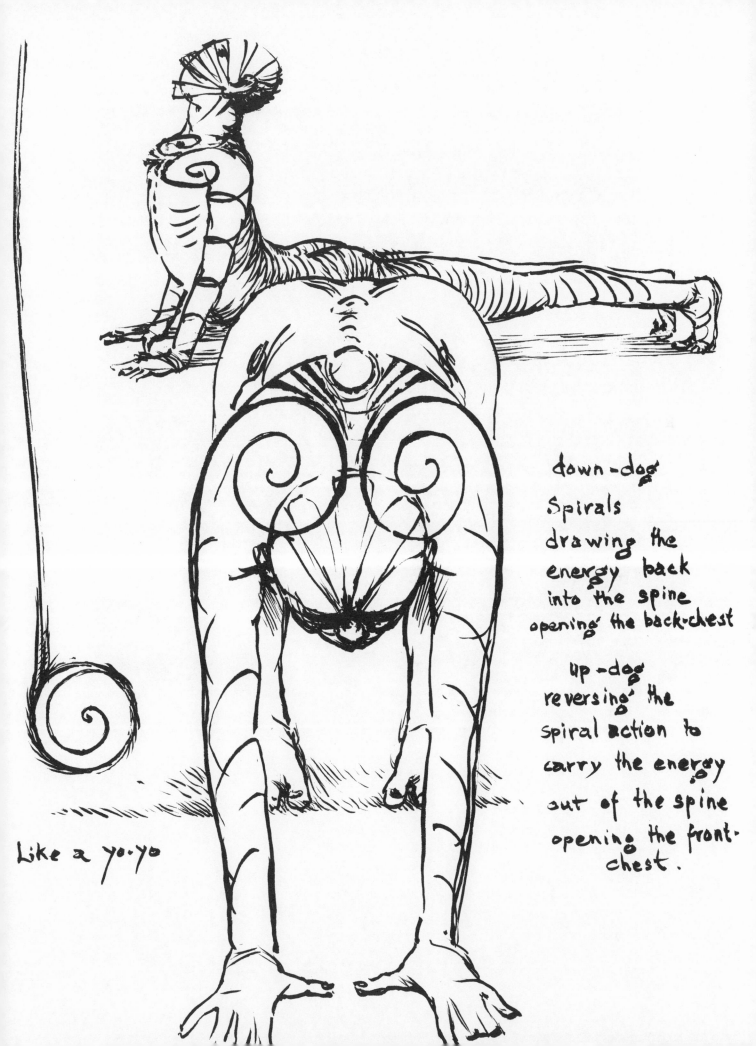

down-dog
Spirals
drawing the
energy back
into the spine
opening the back-chest

up-dog
reversing the
spiral action to
carry the energy
out of the spine
opening the front-
chest.

Like a yo-yo

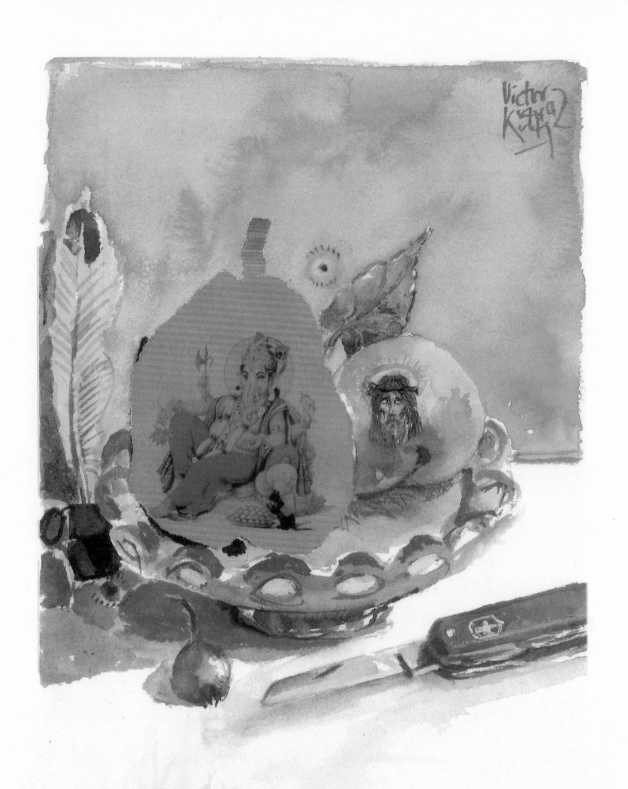

CONSUMERS OF RELIGIONS

We are consumers,
    not growing what we eat.
We buy imported goods from afar.
import religions too...

If you meet the Buddha on the road
                Kill HiM
that will just be a beginning
for now you have to eat
and digest Him.

            listen to what you say
            Hear what your Buddha-mind
            is teaching the listener in you now!

            These teachings,
            no matter how old,
            are a-live,
            they glisten.

I beg you:
free your parrot
from the cage
out into the all absorbing jungle,
            never to come back to you
            and repeat over and over
            things already spoken...

They are almost humans, but are we too far from being animals?

since every living thing finds balance in order to survive, only fools take that for granted.

the Fool

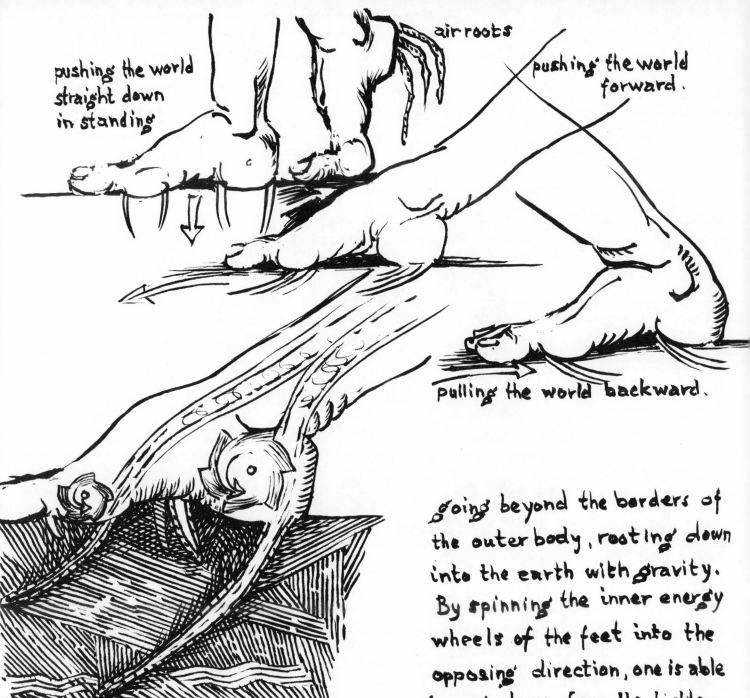

pushing the world straight down in standing

air roots

pushing the world forward.

pulling the world backward.

growing roots down, pumping energy up.

going beyond the borders of the outer body, rooting down into the earth with gravity. By spinning the inner energy wheels of the feet into the opposing direction, one is able to root down from the lighter parts of the ball of heel and front foot and at the same time suck up the earth energy from the existing roots into the inner body.

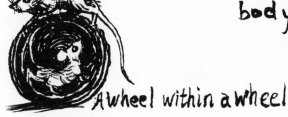

A wheel within a wheel

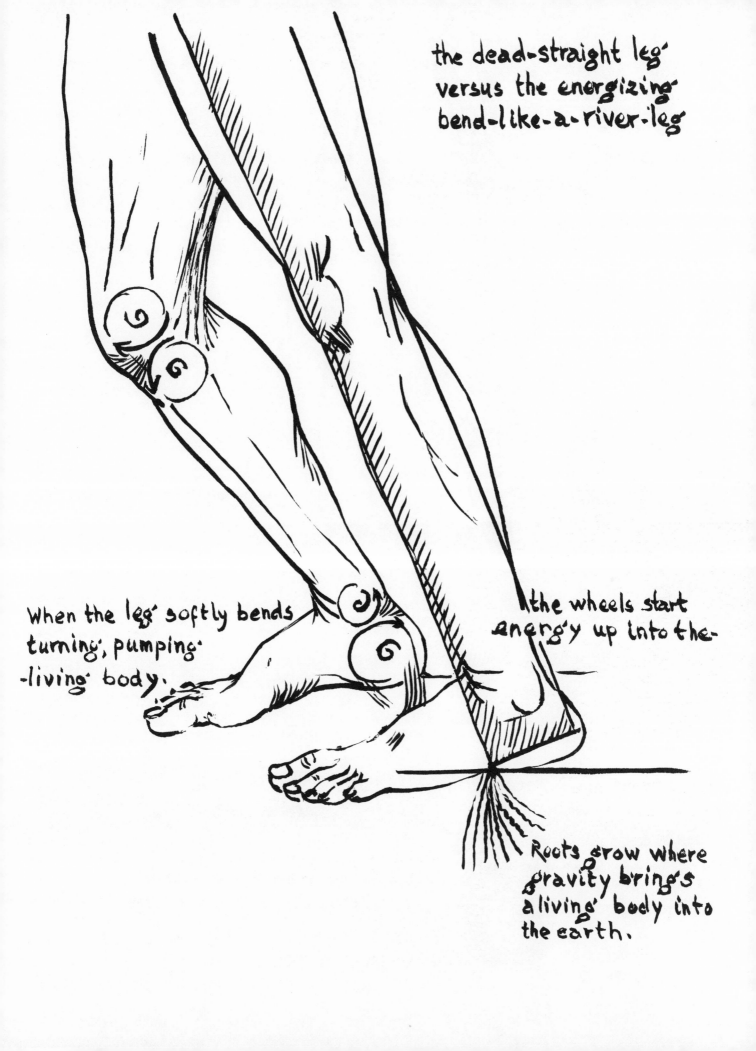

the dead-straight leg
versus the energizing
bend-like-a-river-leg

When the leg softly bends
turning, pumping
-living body.

the wheels start
energy up into the-

Roots grow where
gravity brings
a living body into
the earth.

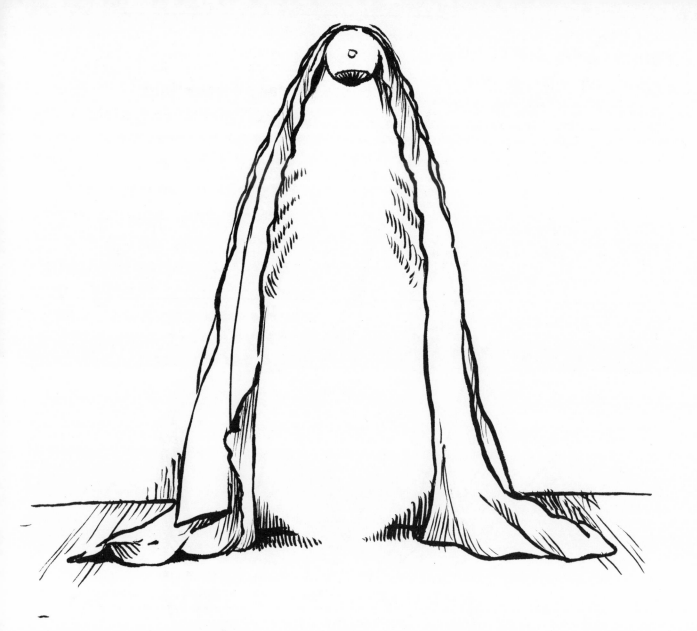

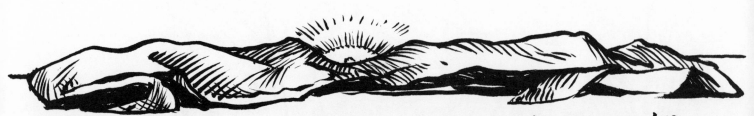

the vision of being far above, dropping with gravity and ease your left
and right garment to earth and becoming centred in your tallness.
Then pour more energy into one side and experience the receptiveness of the earth.

roots are searching
down, bringing the
nourishing earth energy
up, mixing and marrying
the sky.

can you stay well rooted
through your feet
as you move far over
to one side into the
stretching hip and shoulder,
feeling the down pour into
the earth and staying with
that experience, bring the
energy up out of the earth
and let it flow through you
into the opposite side, like
a heavy blanket, sliding off
a horse's back .. ??

inside a Cosmic Egg is life

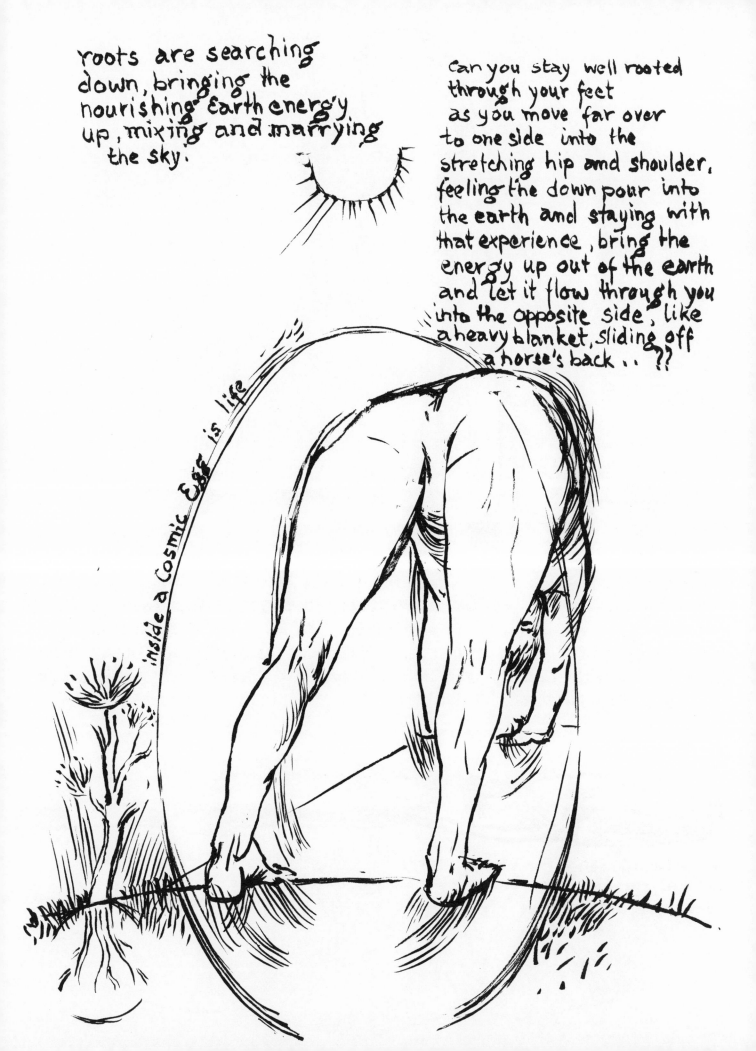

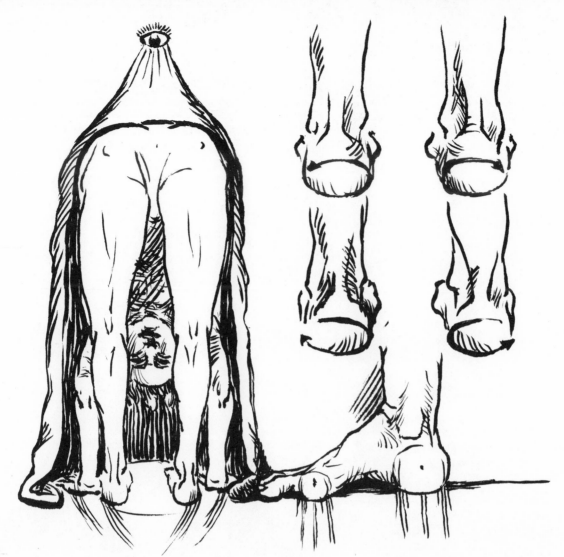

There is a game we play to become aware of the importance of where we put our mind. Once centered in a standing forward-bend, can we relax enough to experience the subtle changes that occur elsewhere; in our legs, pelvis and sacrum, while we massage the earth with our heels, visualising different path ways for the energy-roots to follow.

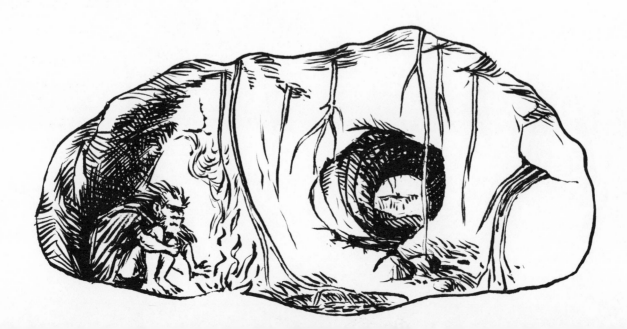

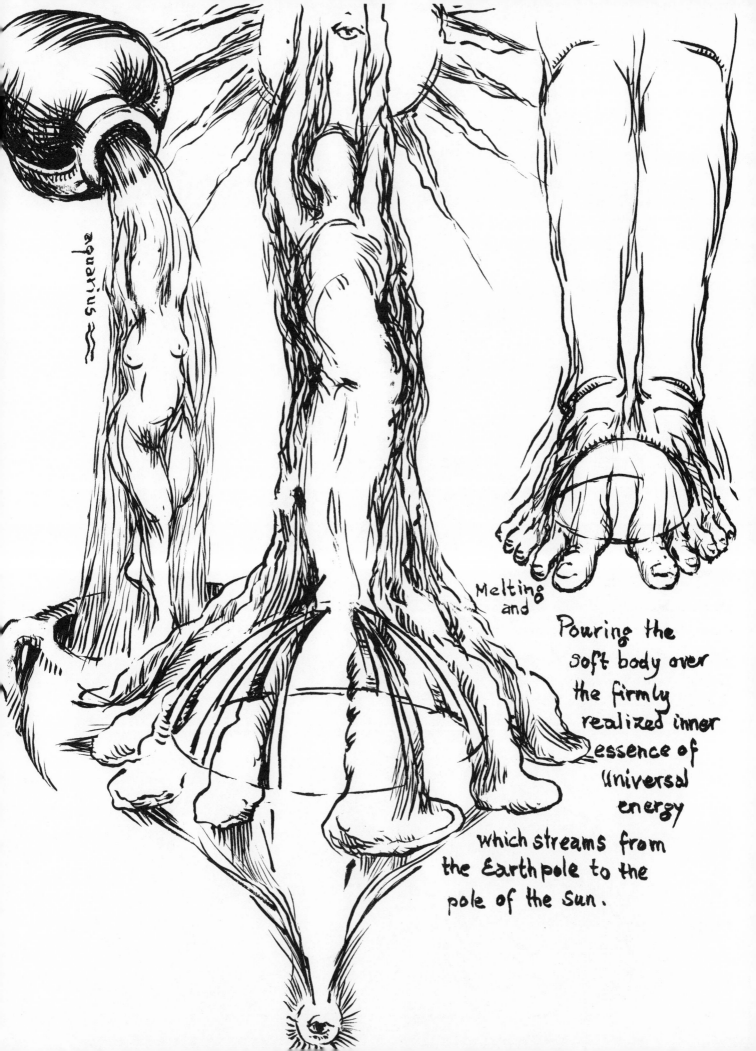

aquarius

Melting
and

Pouring the
soft body over
the firmly
realized inner
essence of
universal
energy

which streams from
the Earthpole to the
pole of the Sun.

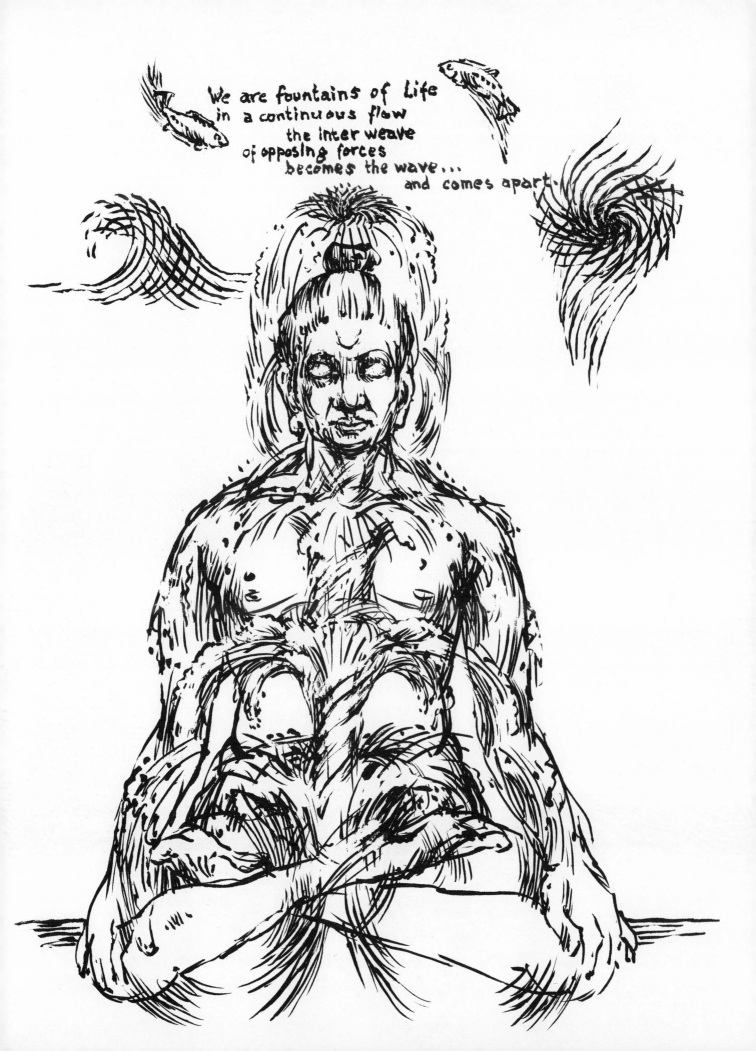

We are fountains of Life
in a continuous flow
    the inter weave
of opposing forces
    becomes the wave...
        and comes apart.

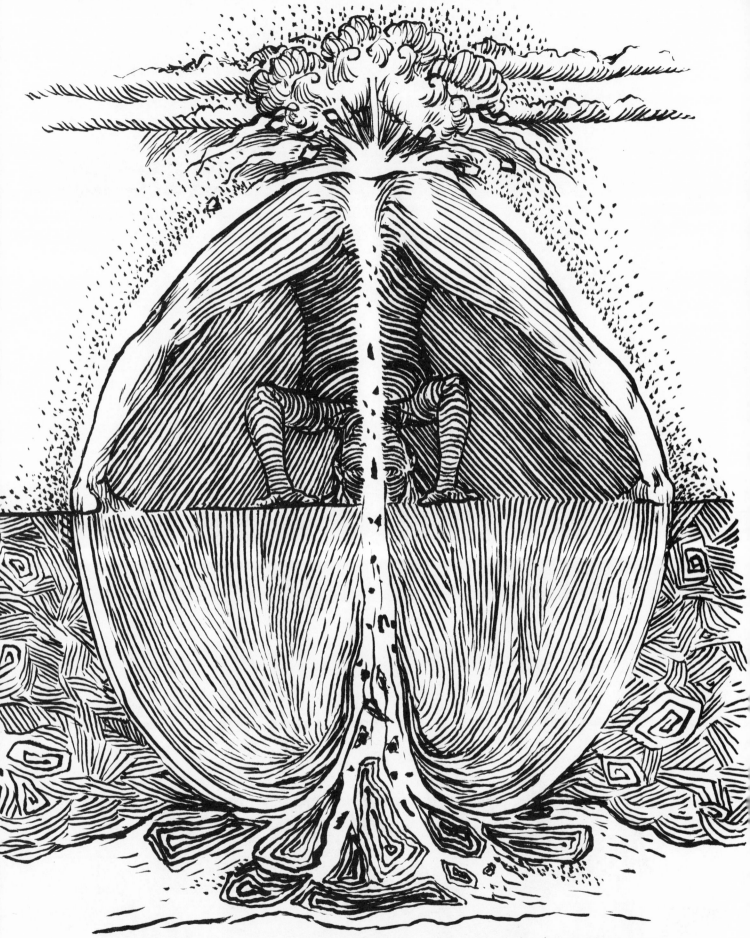

a volcano gets born by sending the upsurging energy from the center down over the outer legs, rooting down from the outer feet deep into the earth, a full circle . . .

returning the energy-stream back
to where it came from.
without changing the fixed position
externally, sucking it up from the weighted
side into the light side that has the tendency
to become uprooted.

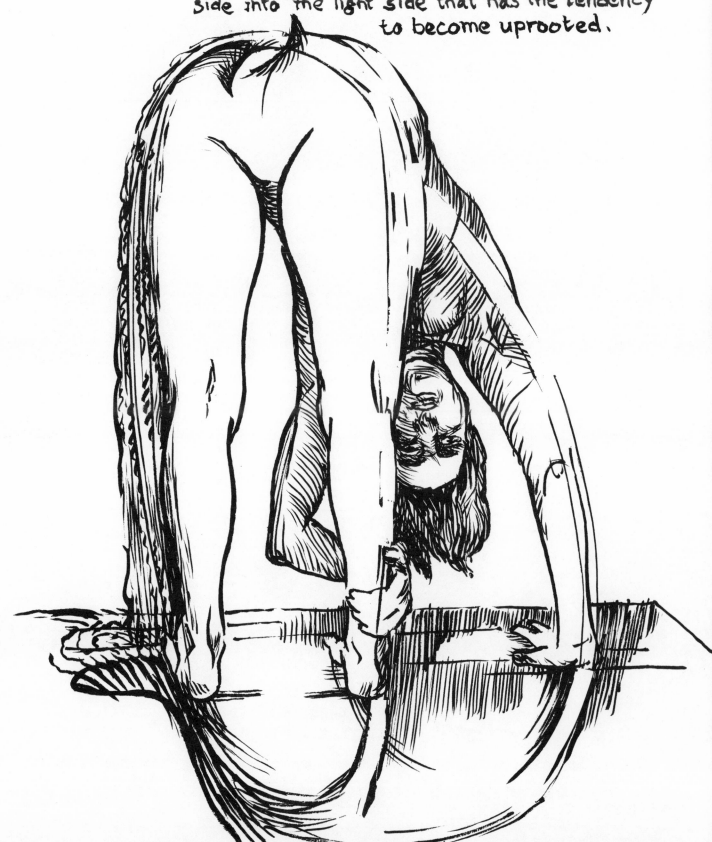

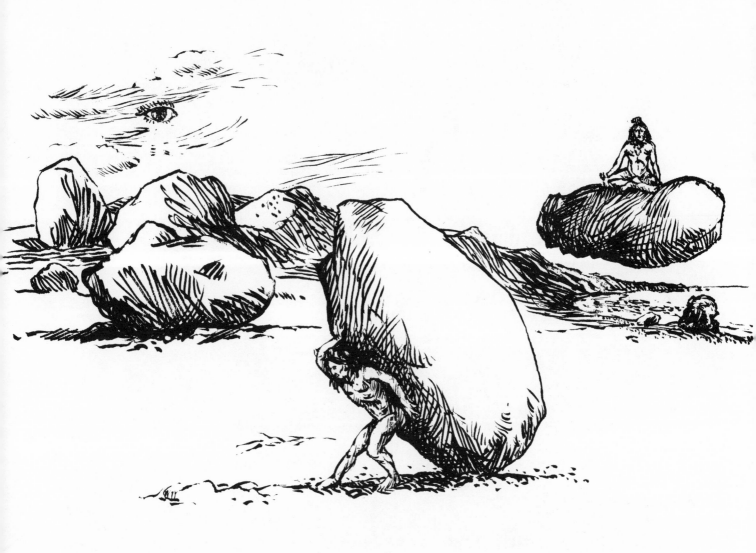

understanding the force   physical force   mental force

Same pose   Same gravity

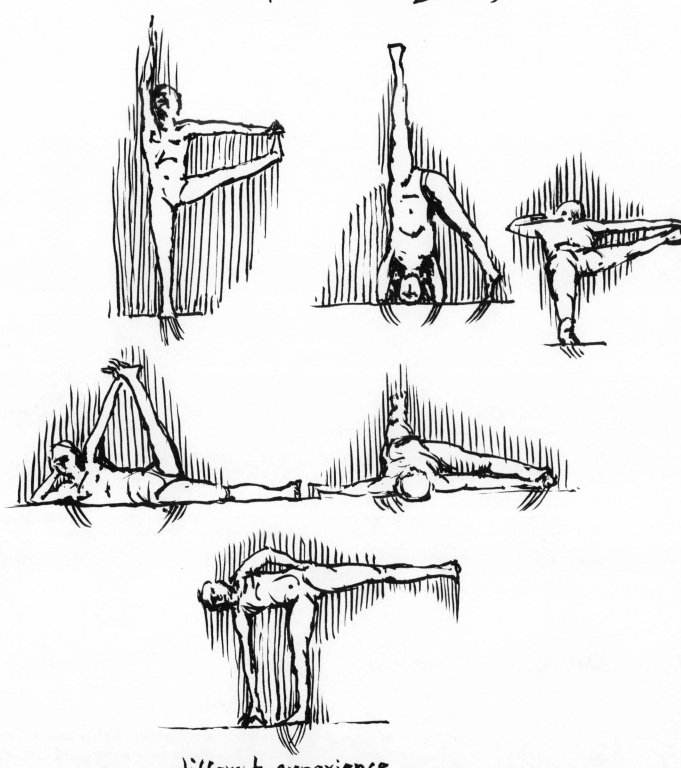

different experience
let all energy come from rooting
floating in the stream of effortlessness.

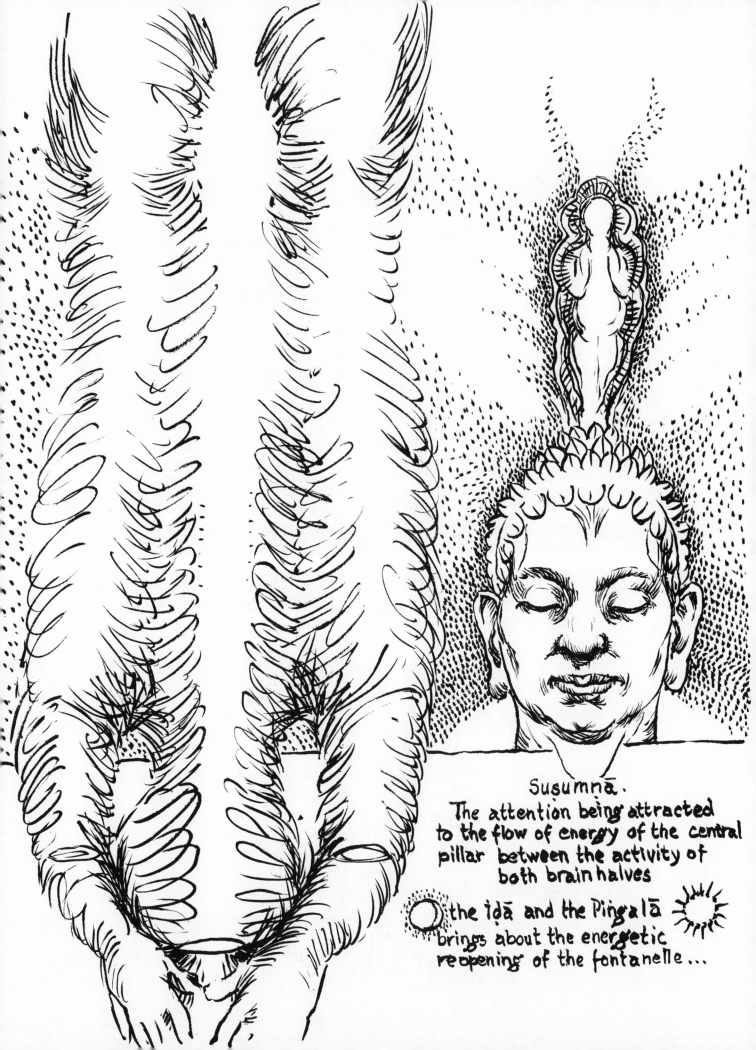

Susumnā.
The attention being attracted
to the flow of energy of the central
pillar between the activity of
both brain halves

the idā and the Pingalā
brings about the energetic
reopening of the fontanelle ...

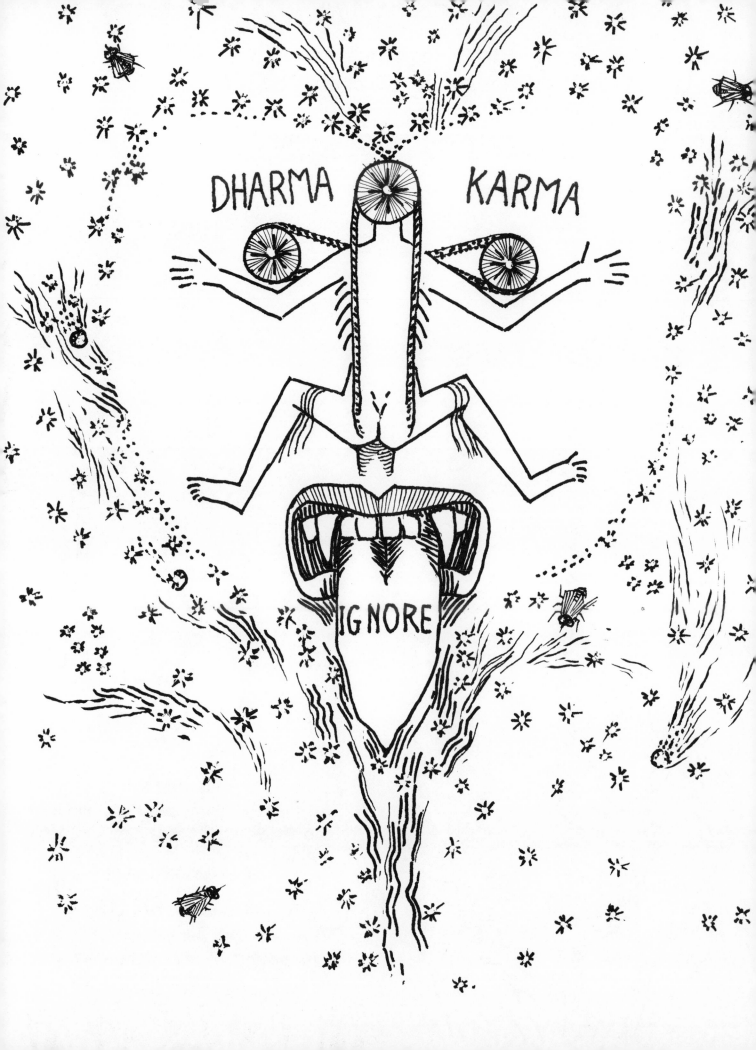

C. spectabilis lightens its load in the hand that frees it –
a movement observed before almost every take off.
(Ronald D. Cave in the National Geographic
Febr 2001 writing about the Jewel Scarabs
of Honduras. After a photo-
graph by David Hawks)

Spreading energy wings
of your pelvic bowl
can change the flow
and shape.

the upward direction
of the energy spiral
created the shape of
your pelvis.

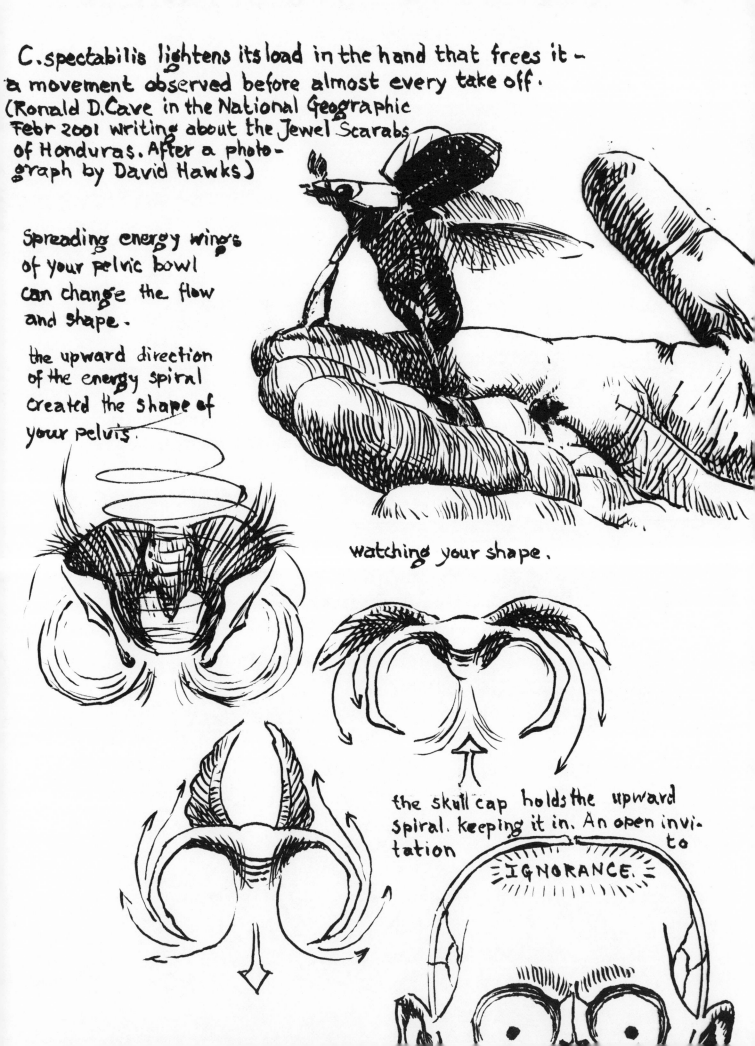

watching your shape.

the skull cap holds the upward
spiral. keeping it in. An open invi-
tation   to
IGNORANCE.

Underneath this
Sleeping beauty
lies a longing lover.

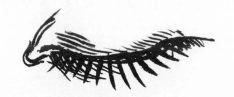

When we have the possibility to know, but we are
unwilling to investigate, we ignore. As soon as the un-
derlying curiosity wakes up, it starts to dissolve and
digest the ignorance, eating it away and transform-
ing it into love. It is only through the love of life, that
we start to understand it. It is only through the love
of our body that we come to know it in an intimate and
personal way, your own unique way, based upon your
taste and love.
    Beneath the body lies the psyche, which connects
to the soul.
    Sit down and open yourself to the many layers of
your being. Open to the joy and just watch the streaming of it all. Allow your fears, that keep your body tightly
closed in a defensive grip, to be digested through
longing for the soul's samadhi, a hidden
hearth deep inside our outward
journey.

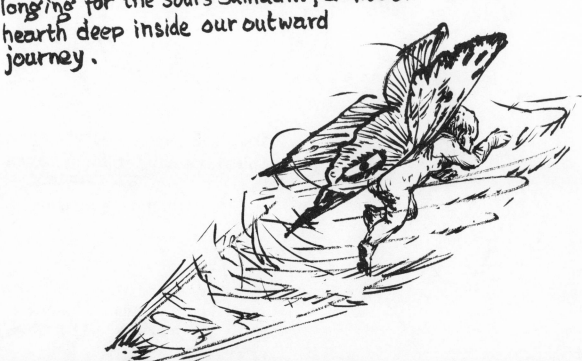

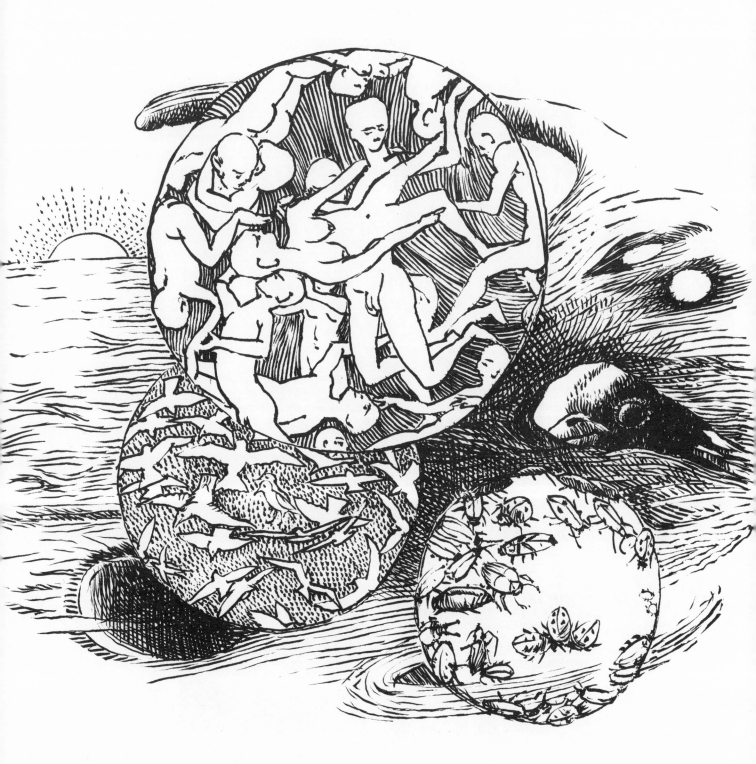

the real life is inside the rotting wood.

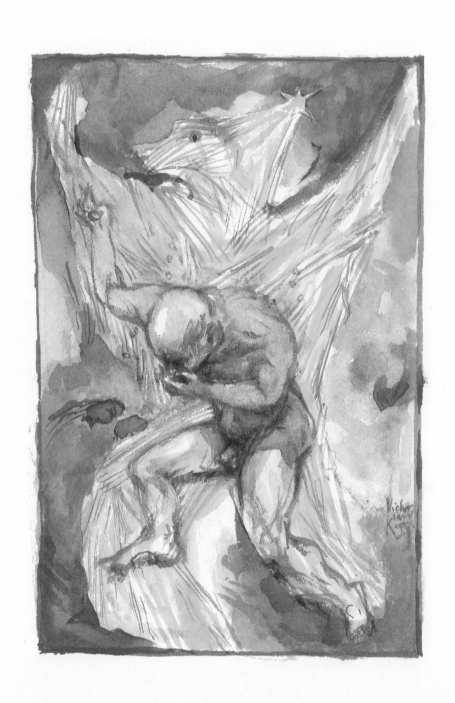

Open up

Unwrap this present
  from its complex soft container,
  born onto the straw that once carried grain.
  his body turned to bread,
  his blood became the wine,
  spread far and wide
  over your dining table.
  When it is all gone
  in the empty space
  remains the presence
  of the maker.
  Feminine teachings
  from the hole inside
  your visible ear
  like the unseen wind passing
  in and out your breathing chest.
      the round shape of the earth
  you stand upon,
  became the arches of your feet,
  your hollow palms
  fold around the nothingness
      you will never catch...
      Open up

Repetition Repetition
Repetition Repetition

Even when you try
to repeat your thoughts,
actions, or in imitating someone else,
you will discover subtle changes
which deform or even reshape the image.
For nothing will ever remain the same under the ever changing
light in this living world. On the other hand, we tend to hold on
tight to our form with a skin that separates us from others and
our environment, keeping us from losing our identity...
  WHY DO YOU STICK TO YOUR ROUTINE?

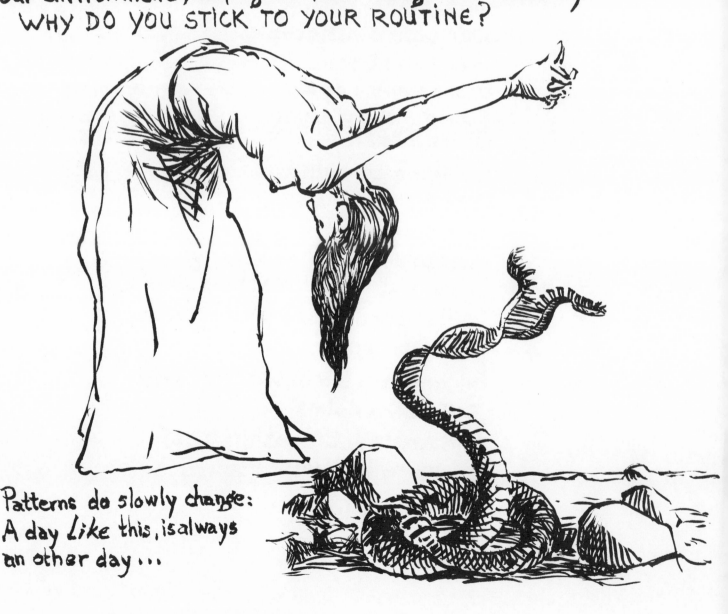

Patterns do slowly change:
A day *Like* this, is always
an other day...

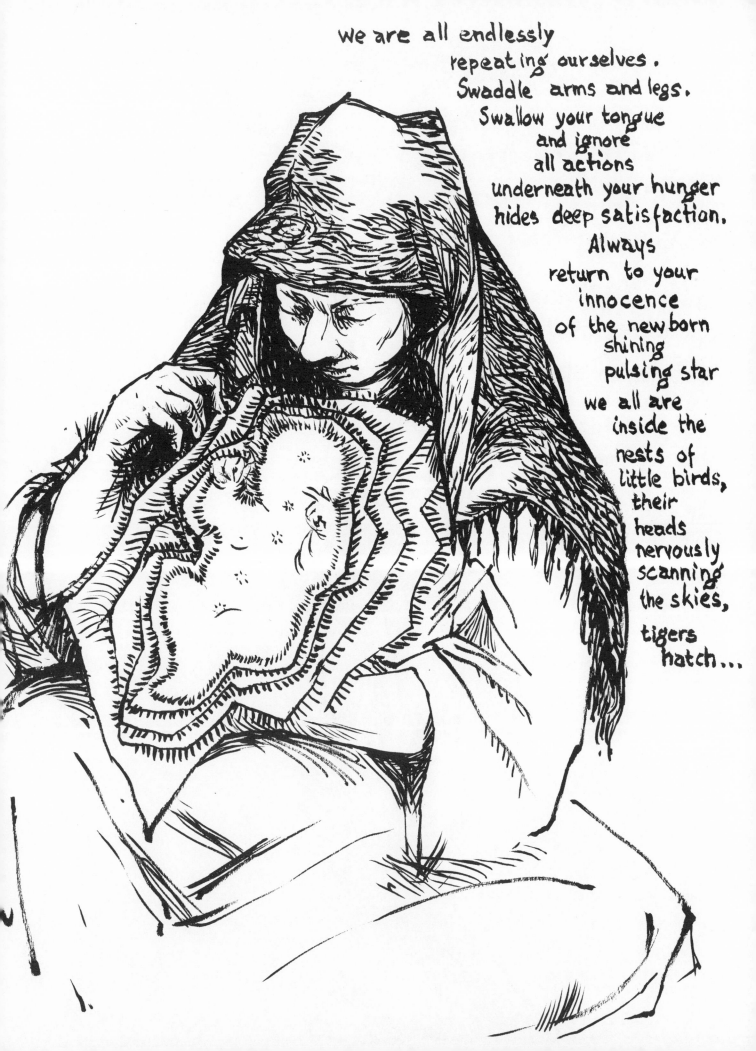

we are all endlessly
repeating ourselves.
Swaddle arms and legs.
Swallow your tongue
and ignore
all actions
underneath your hunger
hides deep satisfaction.
Always
return to your
innocence
of the newborn
shining
pulsing star
we all are
inside the
nests of
little birds,
their
heads
nervously
scanning
the skies,
tigers
hatch...

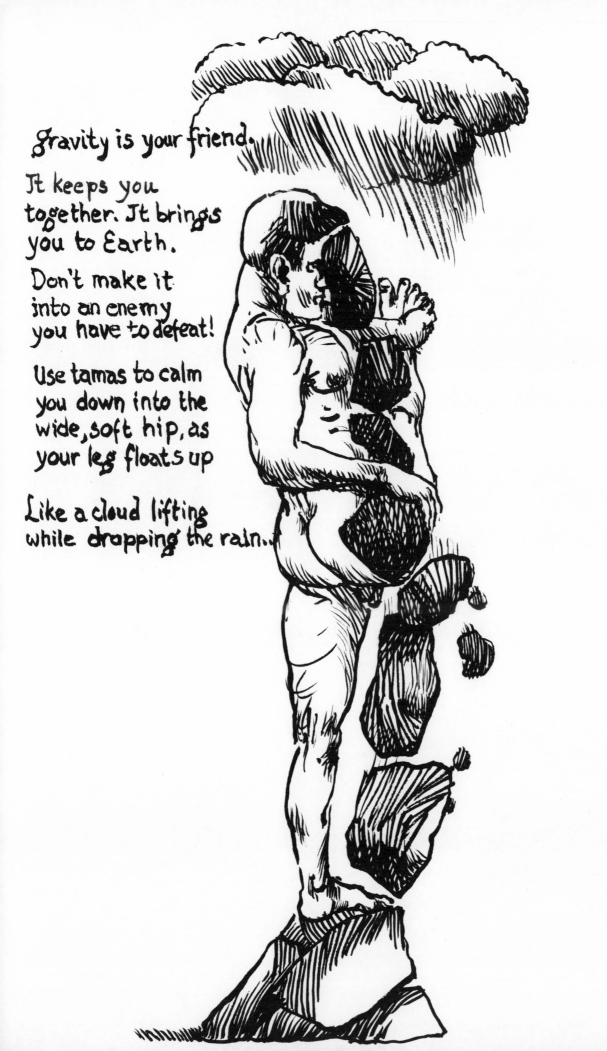

Gravity is your friend.

It keeps you together. It brings you to Earth.

Don't make it into an enemy you have to defeat!

Use tamas to calm you down into the wide, soft hip, as your leg floats up

Like a cloud lifting while dropping the rain...

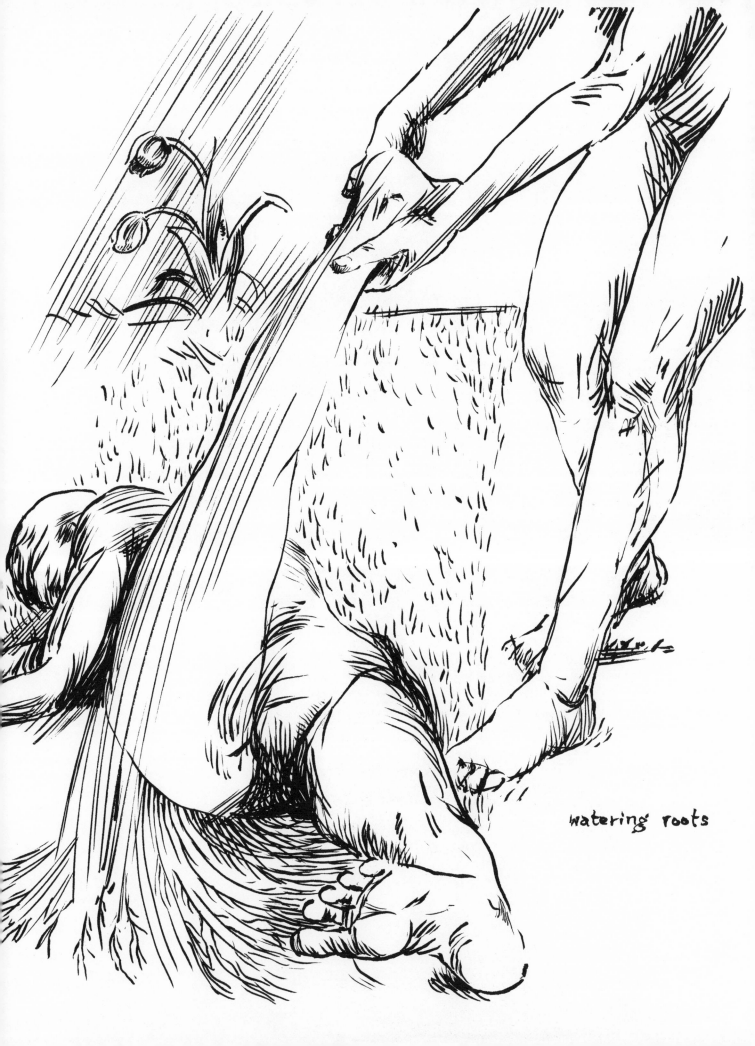

watering roots

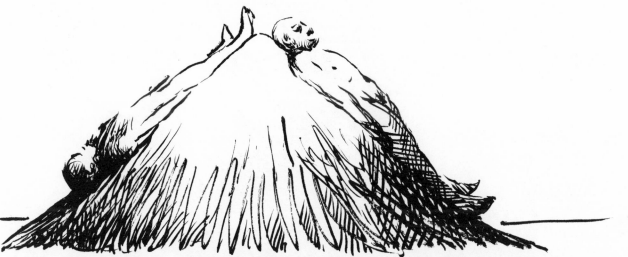

By invoking the Earth to tilt, so it becomes a hill
on which we lie in different positions, head down-hill
or head up-hill, the hilltop to our right and valley below
on our left, or the other way around, we will be able to
experience the opening and closing of body areas
without any physical effort from our side

and inside the nostrils
the breath will touch
different areas too!

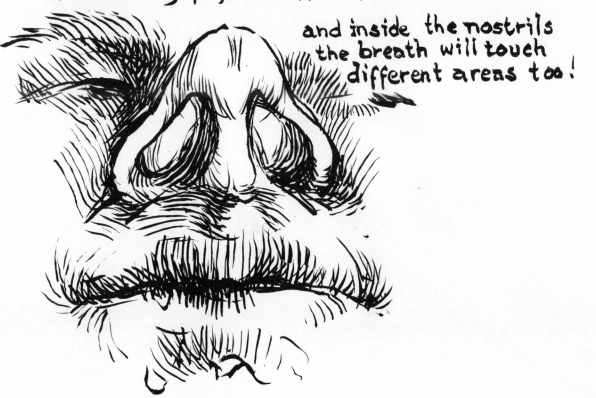

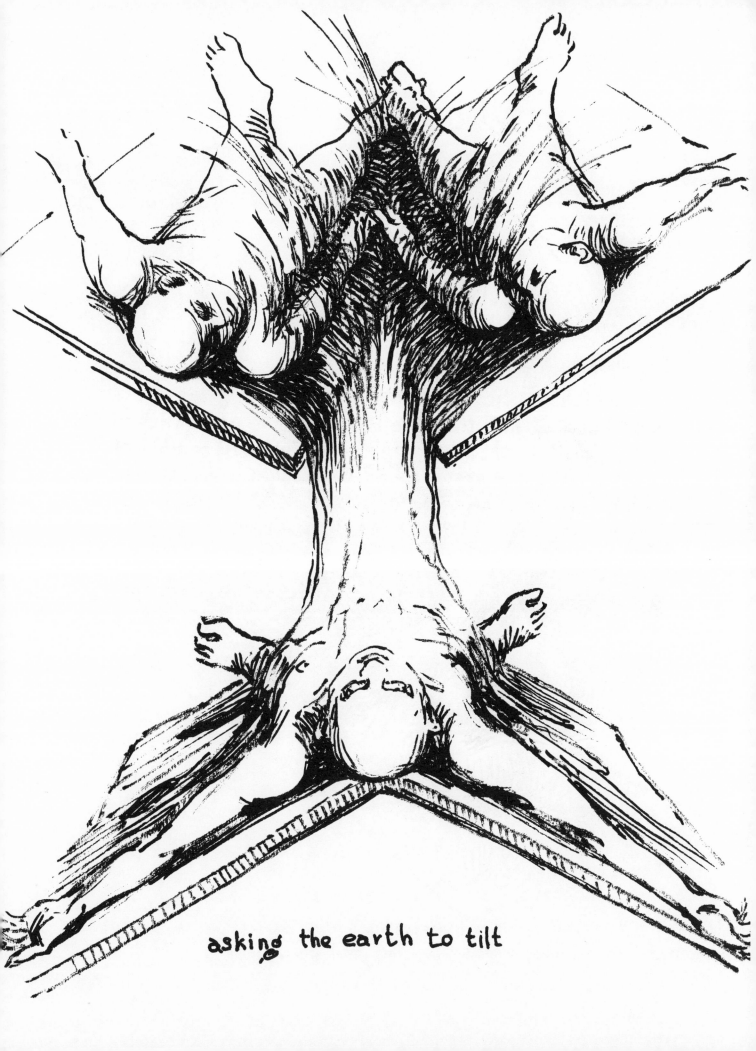

asking the earth to tilt

Yoga East - Yoga West

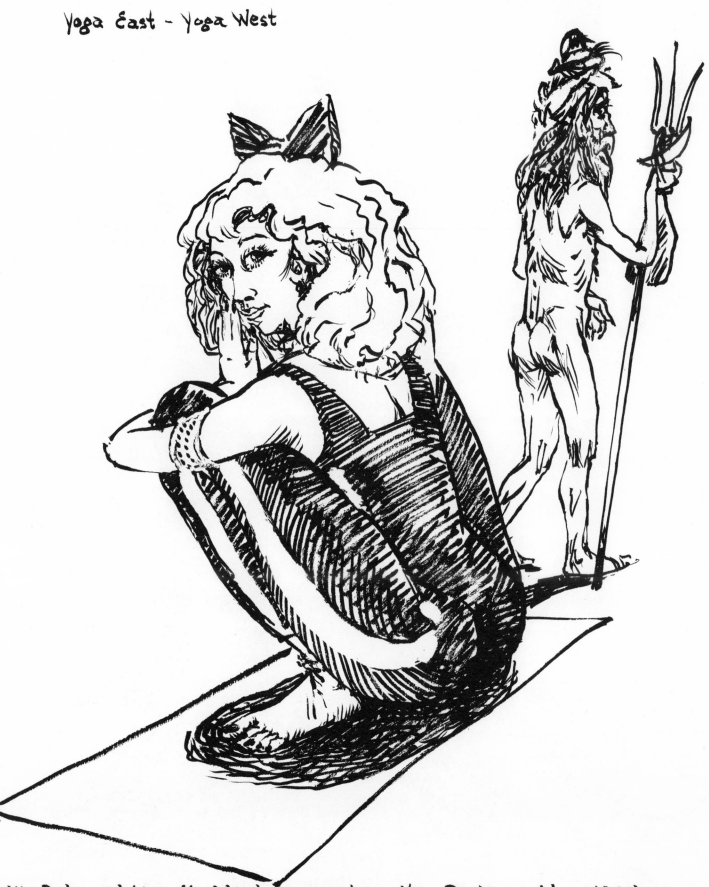

While Baba rid himself of his last posessions, Yoga Barbie got herself into a new stretch outfit and bought the new improved purple mat.

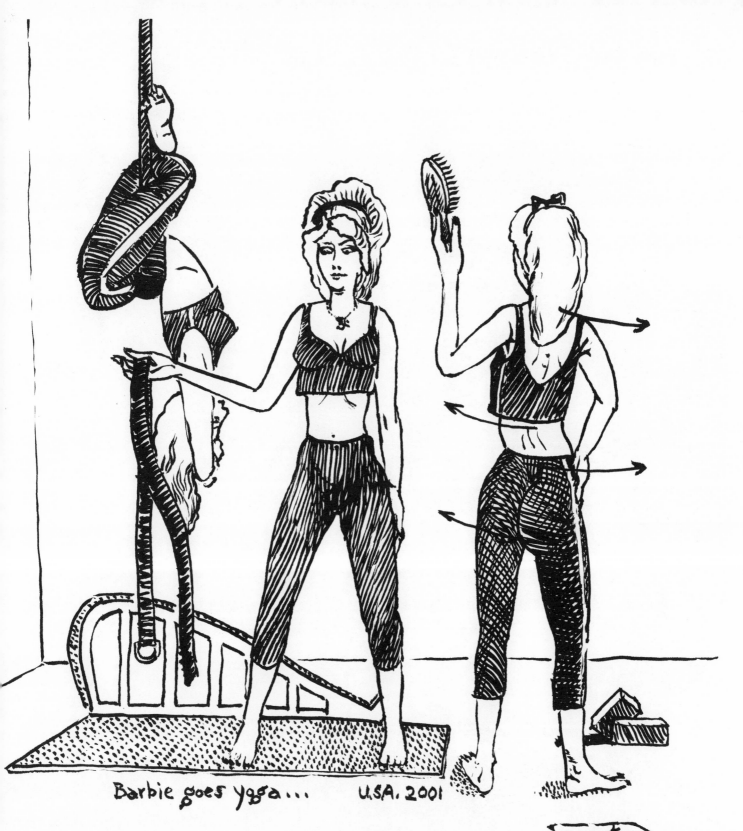

Barbie goes yoga...   U.S.A. 2001

for a more flexible
body, try to move your perineum
to the left, as the top pelvis
moves to the right, the bottom ribs
to the left, as the shoulders move to
the right.

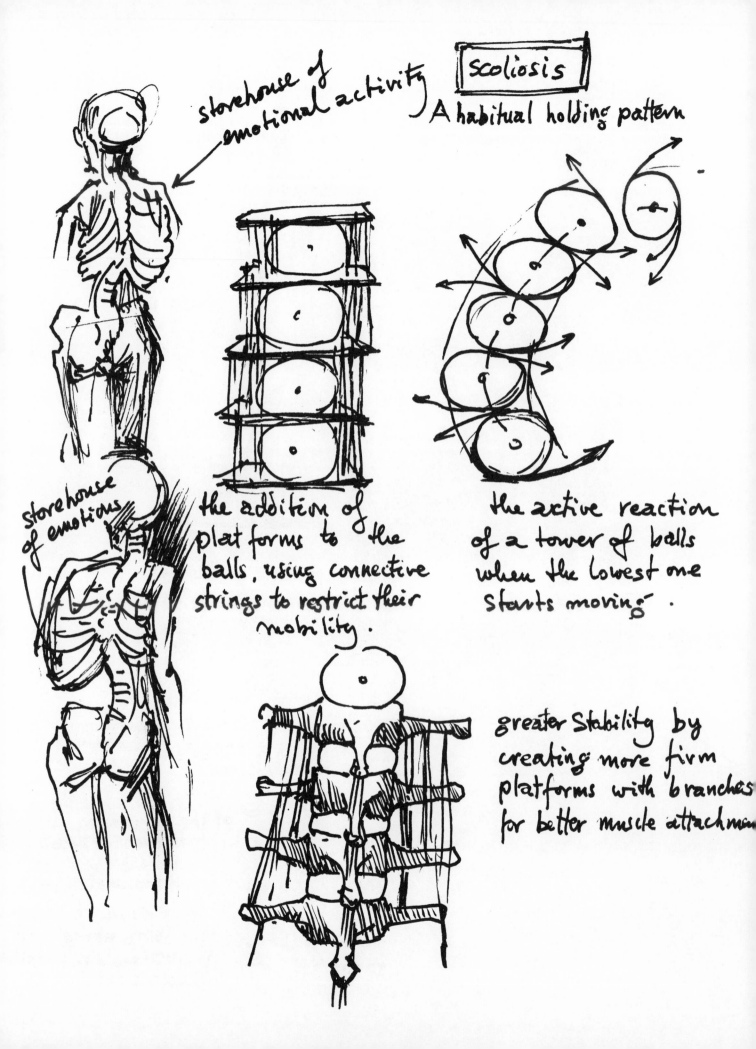

storehouse of
emotional activity

Scoliosis
A habitual holding pattern

storehouse
of emotions

the addition of
platforms to the
balls, using connective
strings to restrict their
mobility.

the active reaction
of a tower of balls
when the lowest one
starts moving.

greater stability by
creating more firm
platforms with branches
for better muscle attachment

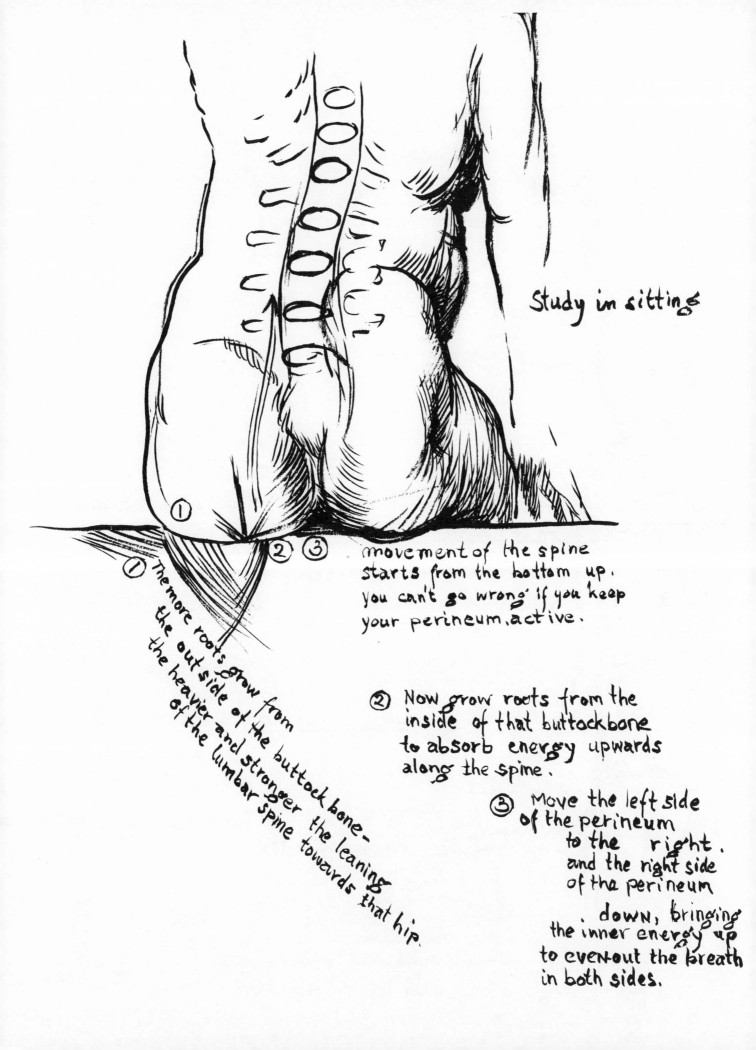

Study in sitting

movement of the spine
starts from the bottom up.
you can't go wrong if you keep
your perineum active.

② Now grow roots from the
inside of that buttockbone
to absorb energy upwards
along the spine.

③ Move the left side
of the perineum
to the right.
and the right side
of the perineum

down, bringing
the inner energy up
to even out the breath
in both sides.

① The more roots grow from
the outside of the buttock bone -
the heavier and stronger the leaning
of the lumbar spine towards that hip.

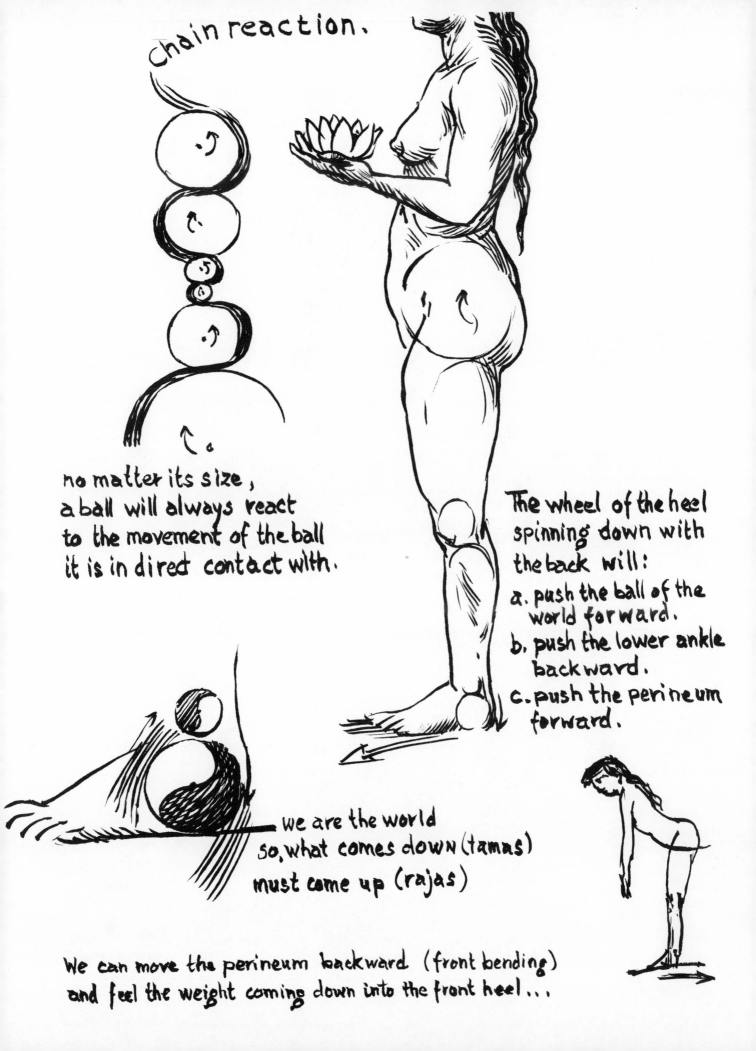

chain reaction.

no matter its size,
a ball will always react
to the movement of the ball
it is in direct contact with.

The wheel of the heel
spinning down with
the back will:
a. push the ball of the
world forward.
b. push the lower ankle
backward.
c. push the perineum
forward.

we are the world
so, what comes down (tamas)
must come up (rajas)

We can move the perineum backward (front bending)
and feel the weight coming down into the front heel...

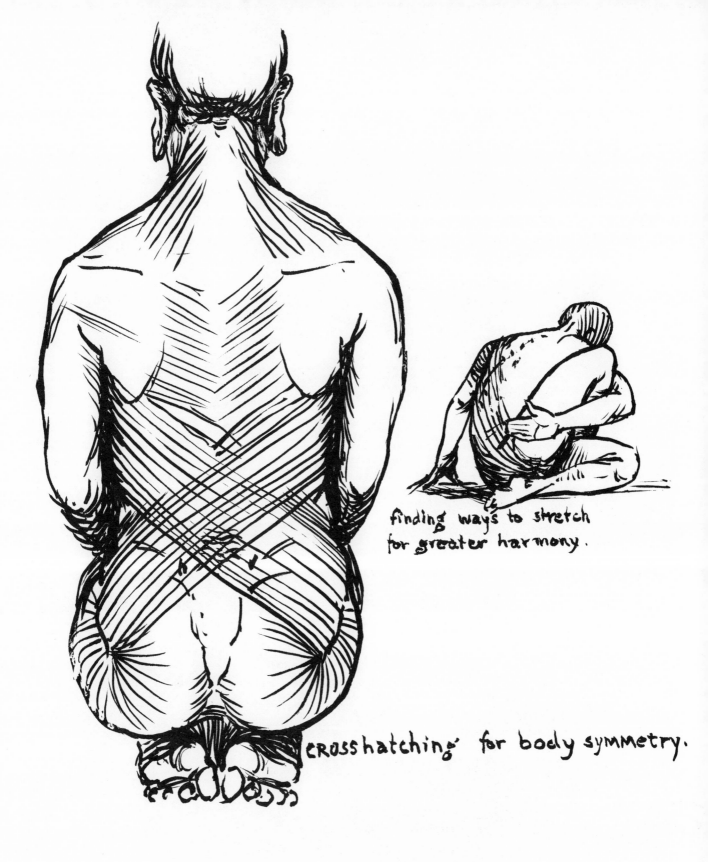

finding ways to stretch
for greater harmony.

crosshatching for body symmetry.

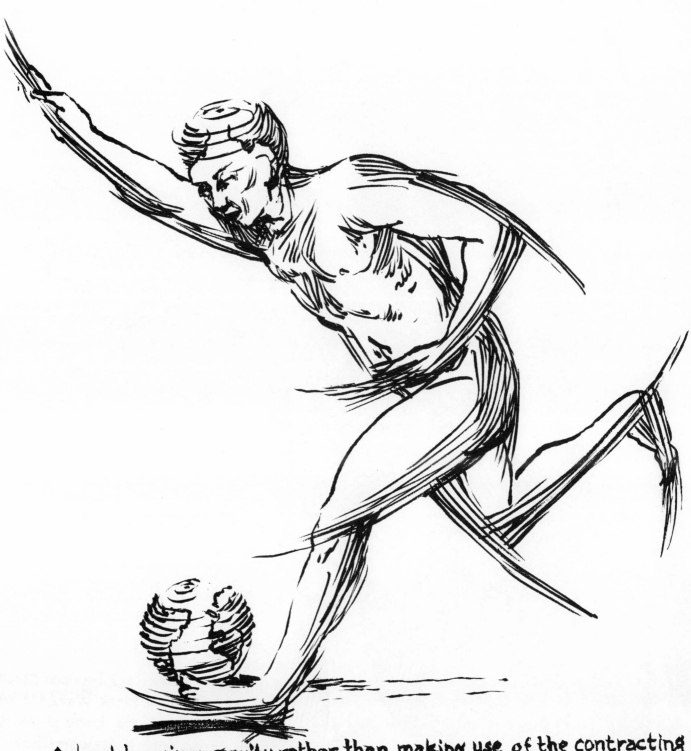

Extend by using gravity rather than making use of the contracting force of muscle strength. It will create more body space in all joints, avoiding wear and tear as you play the world game

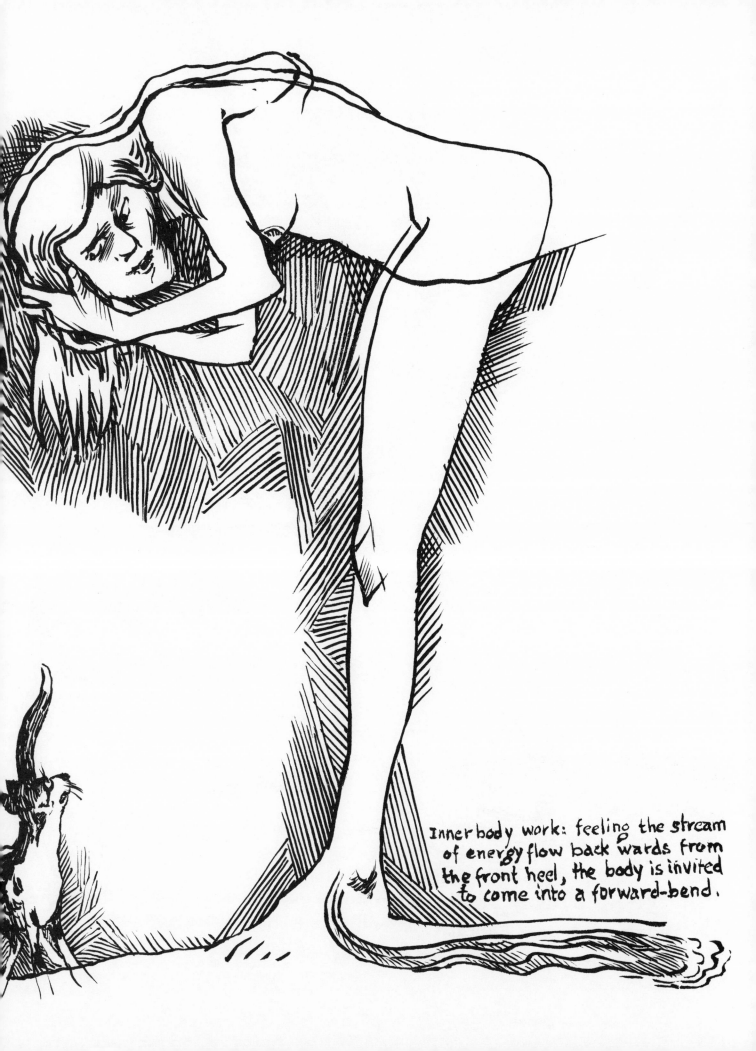

Innerbody work: feeling the stream of energy flow backwards from the front heel, the body is invited to come into a forward-bend.

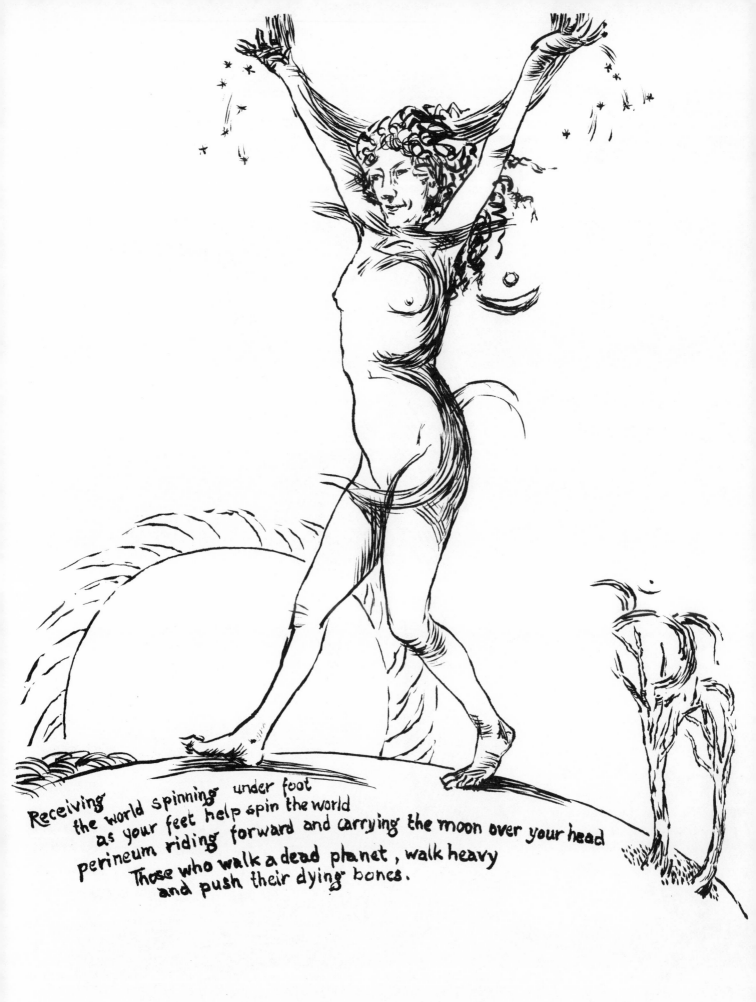

Receiving
  the world spinning under foot
    as your feet help spin the world
perineum riding forward and carrying the moon over your head
  Those who walk a dead planet, walk heavy
    and push their dying bones.

On walking...

    Try many different ways of walking
over and into the earth.
Walk from different areas too;
① following the head like a net
                 catching butterflies.

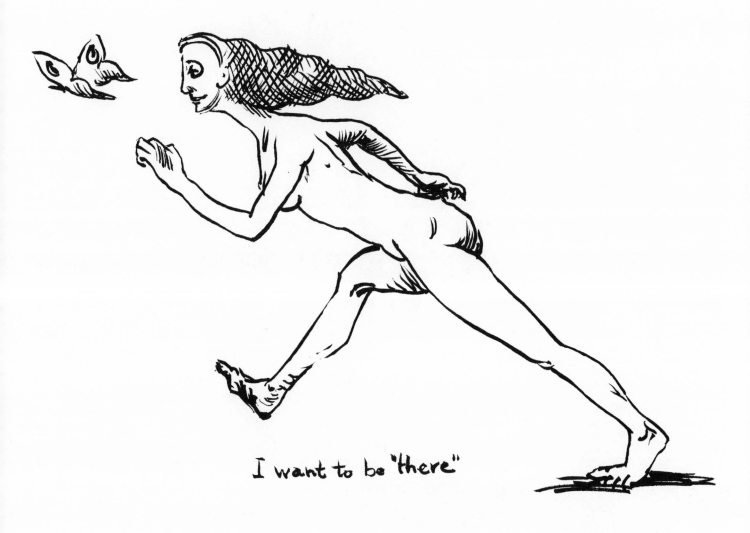

I want to be "there"

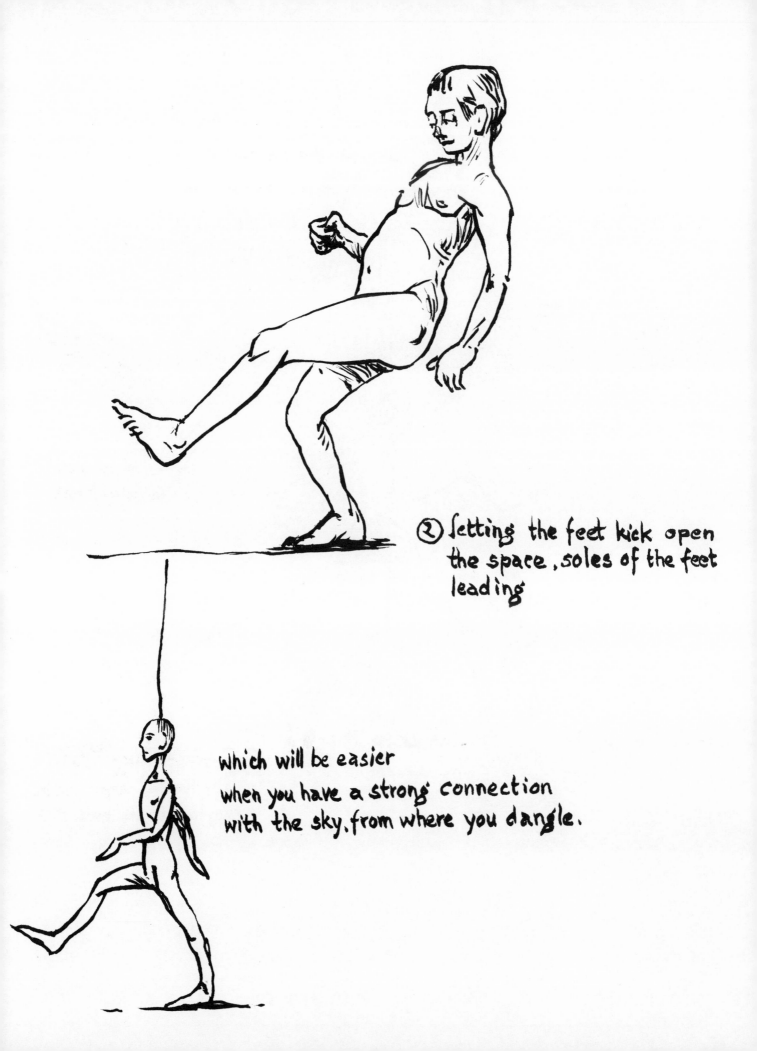

② letting the feet kick open
the space, soles of the feet
leading

which will be easier
when you have a strong connection
with the sky, from where you dangle.

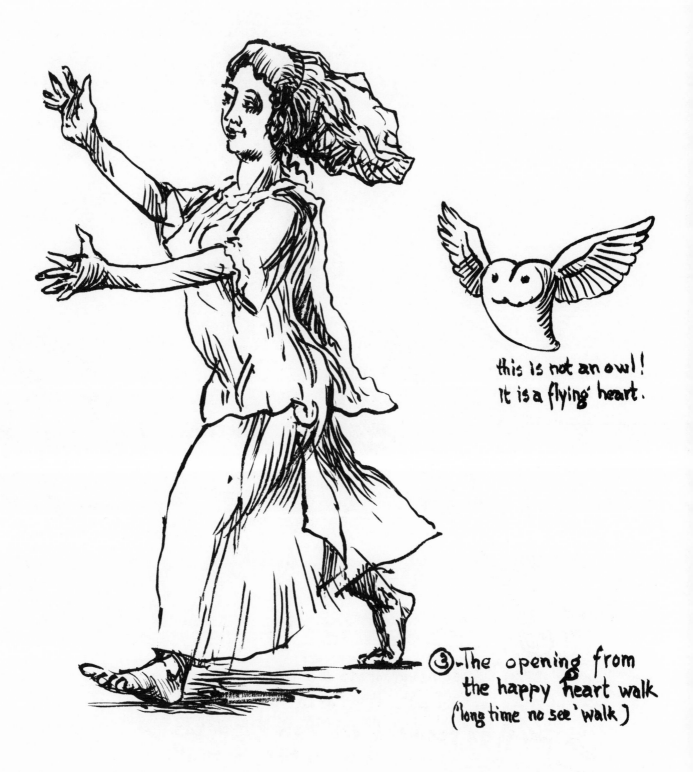

this is not an owl!
It is a flying heart.

③ The opening from
the happy heart walk
('long time no see' walk)

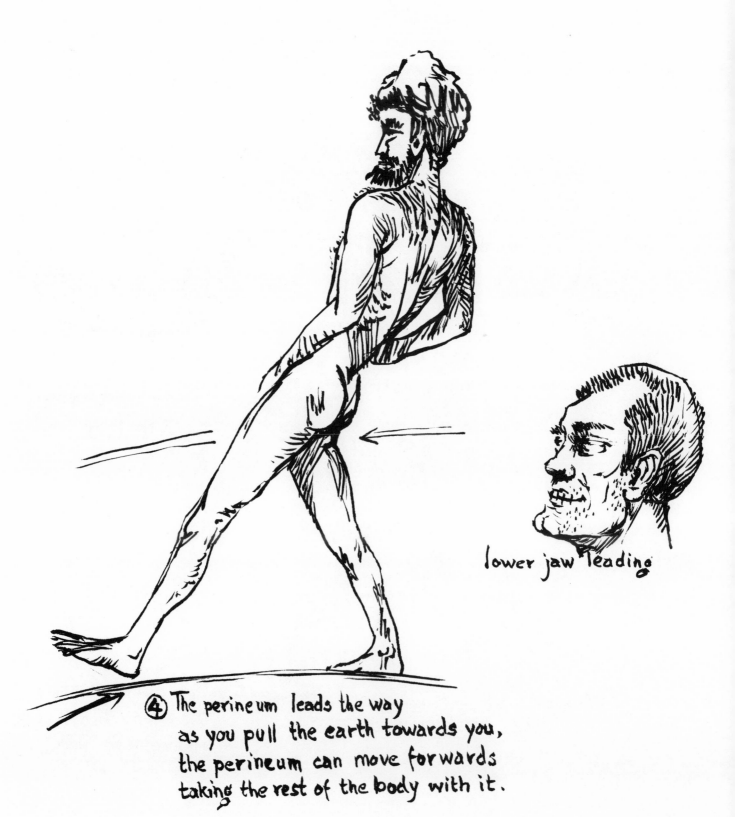

lower jaw leading

④ The perineum leads the way
as you pull the earth towards you,
the perineum can move forwards
taking the rest of the body with it.

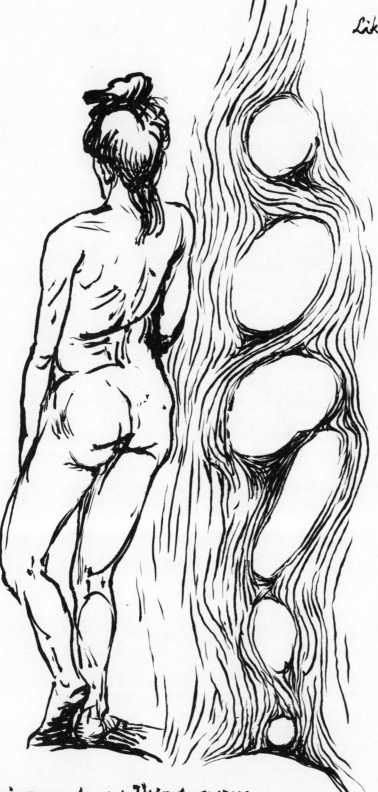

Like Rocks in a mountain stream

The Perineum in walking, sways
   into the right inner leg
   into the left inner leg
which, if it moves freely,
causes the whole body to stream.

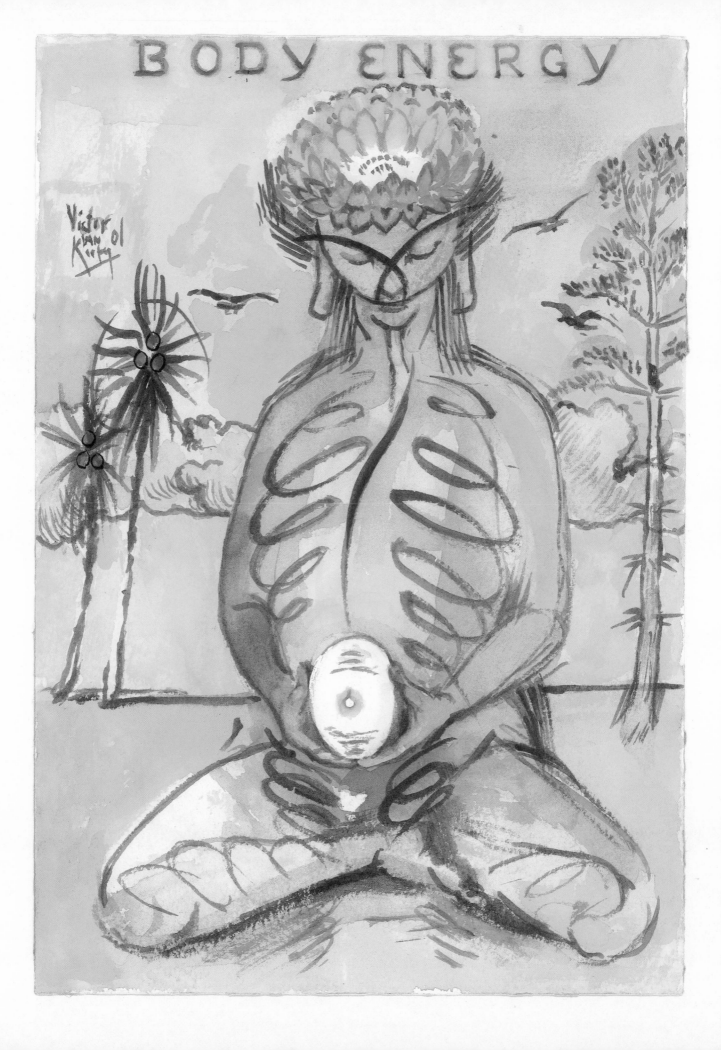

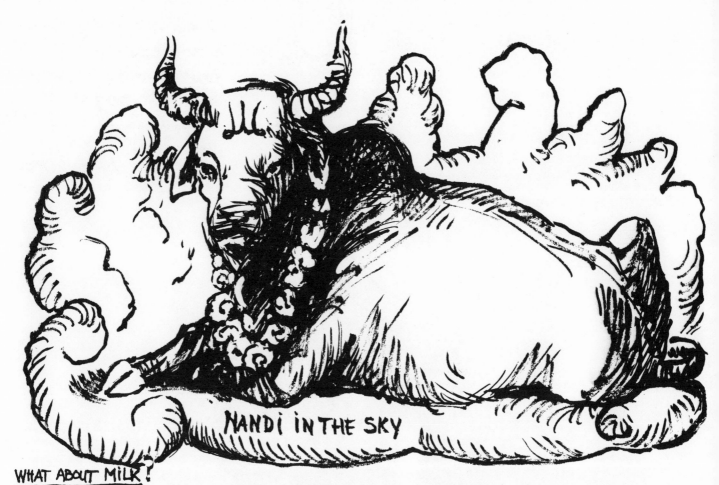

NANDI IN THE SKY

WHAT ABOUT MILK?

When J poured milk into our Chai, Dirk suddenly remarked that he had heard of the theory that aslong as you drink milk, you will never grow up! For sure it is a baby food and given before we can take in any other foods. It makes the small body grow fast, with lots of calcium for developing bones.

I was told, in my Macro-biotic days, that, if you drink cow's milk as a teenager you will grow tall, as the calves do, with far too heavy bones, since you become what you eat!"

In India cow's milk-butter-yoghurt-cheese-all play an important role in the feeding of the people. J met the Milk-Saint in Nepal, a tiny guy with a mass of dread locks falling all around him onto the floor of his dark hut. All he drank was milk. And then there are the Gopies, the milk maids with the butter stealing Krishna and Shiva's vehicle, the bull Nandi.

In India the cow is holy, so the milk transforms into higher consciousness. The body grows and at a certain point does not need all that calcium. It throws it out, or transcends it into spiritual growth if you are willing to elevate the cow and are willing to open up to the spiritual levels of existence. Your body-mind is naturally intelligent, so open up to it and do not just grow up and live with hardened beliefs, but stay in the learning mode of baby Krishna.

I have news for you:

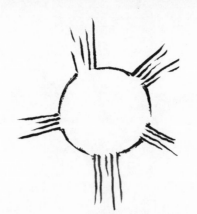

There is nothing new
to be discovered.
You can only discover
what already is and
present it in an original
clear way
or hide it deep under
confusion.

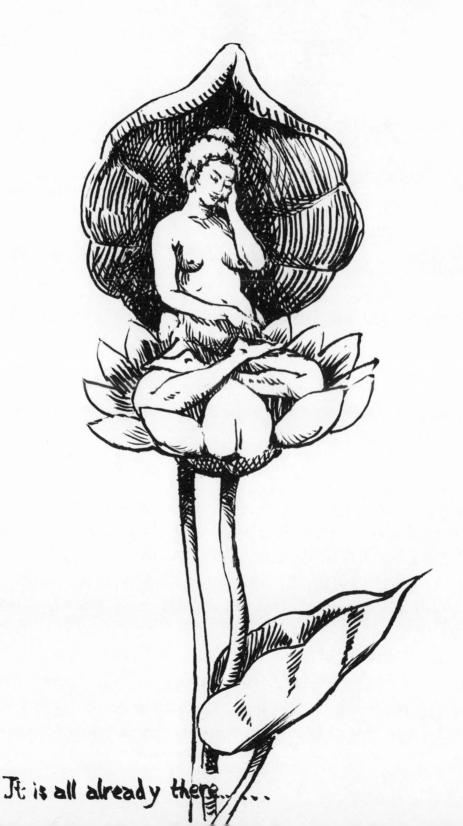

It is all already there......

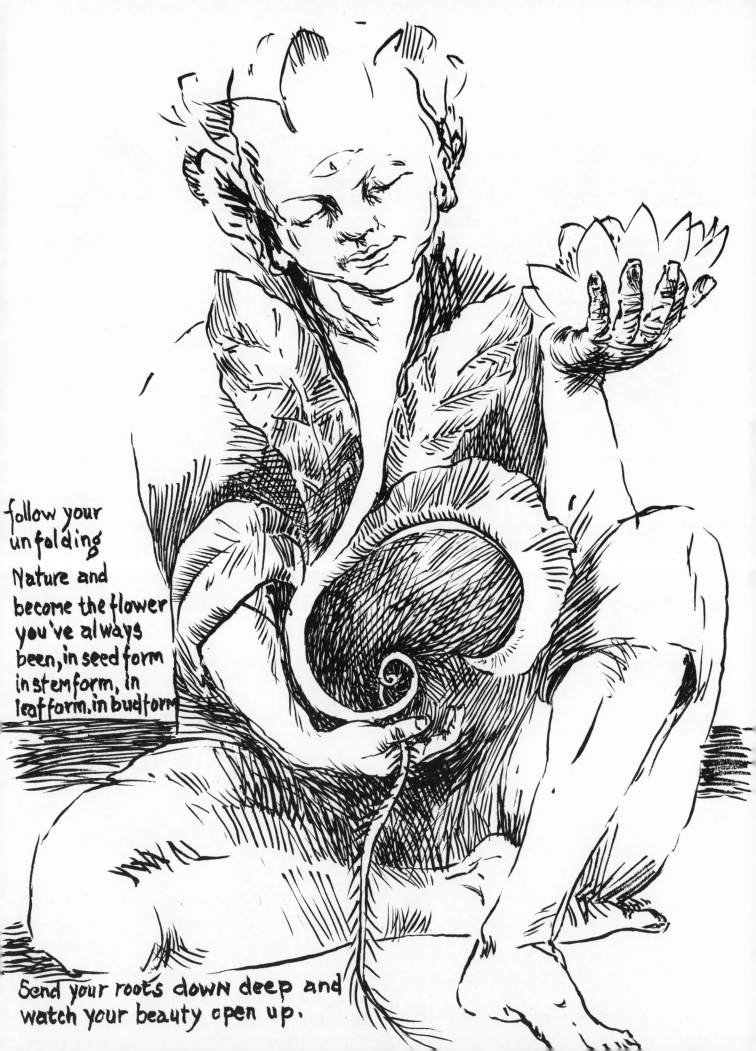

follow your
unfolding
Nature and
become the flower
you've always
been, in seed form
in stem form, in
leaf form, in bud form

Send your roots down deep and
watch your beauty open up.

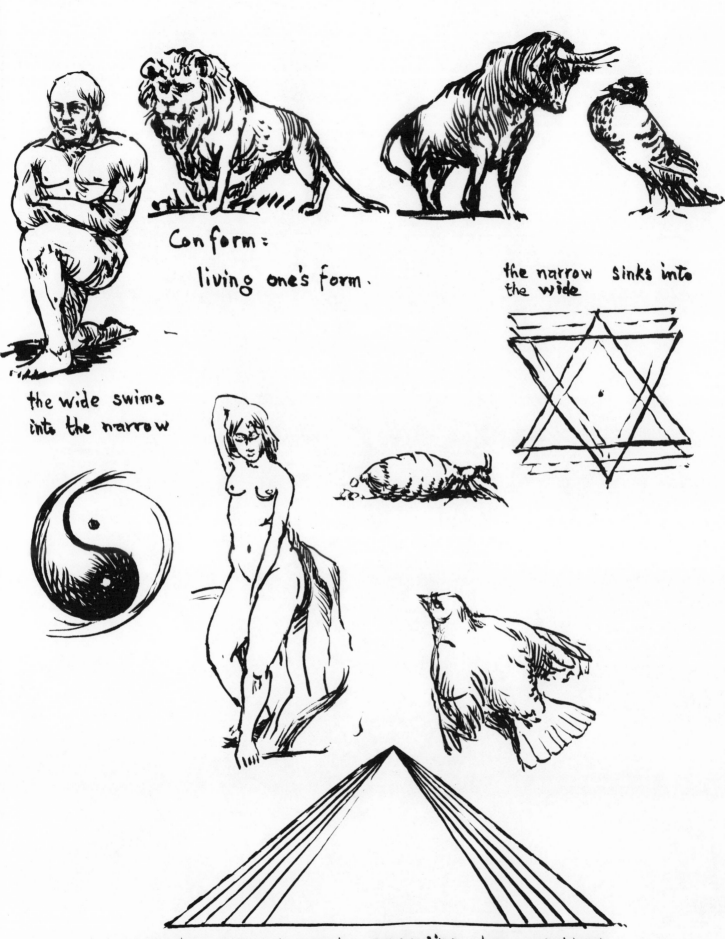

Conform:

living one's form.

the narrow sinks into the wide

the wide swims into the narrow

2 Sides of the triangle: masculine : top-pointing
feminine : base-opening

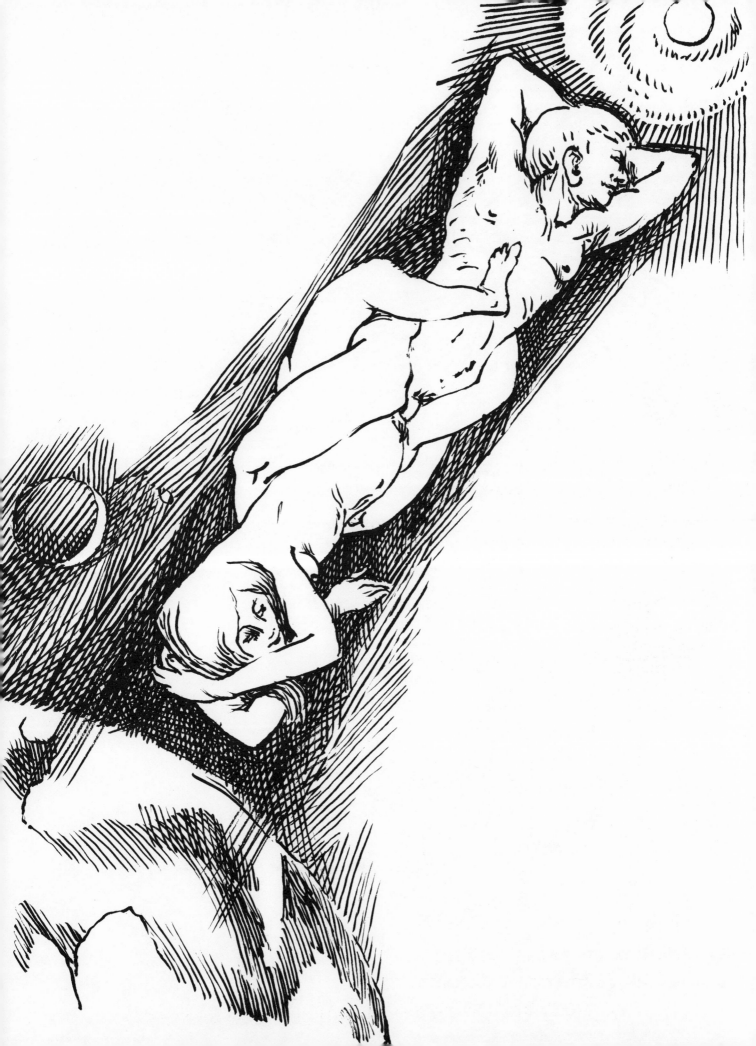

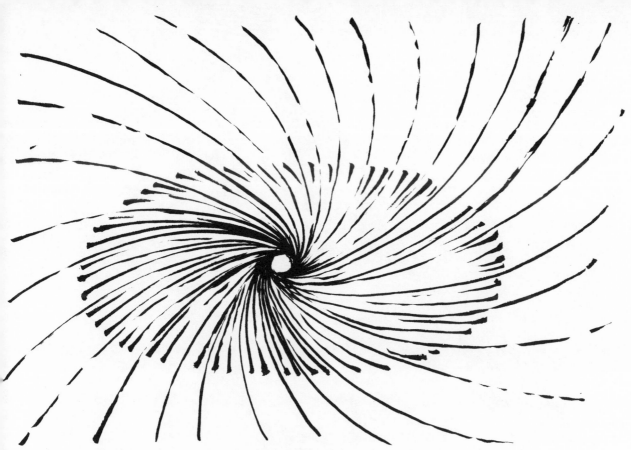

The outer body is a meeting place between
inhalation and exhalation,
between absorption and radiation,
between rajas and tamas.
The skin is a creation of dual action.

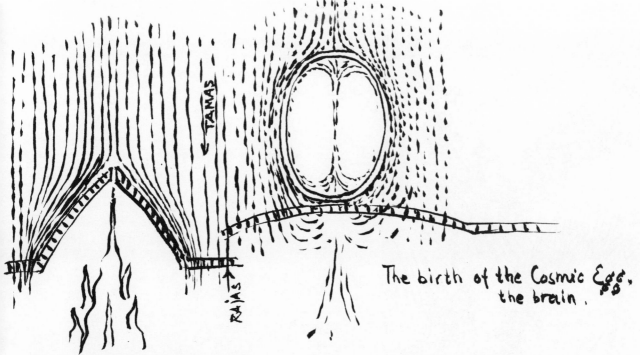

The birth of the Cosmic Egg,
the brain.

the birth of a volcano
a pyramid, an onion and the dome.

What we see 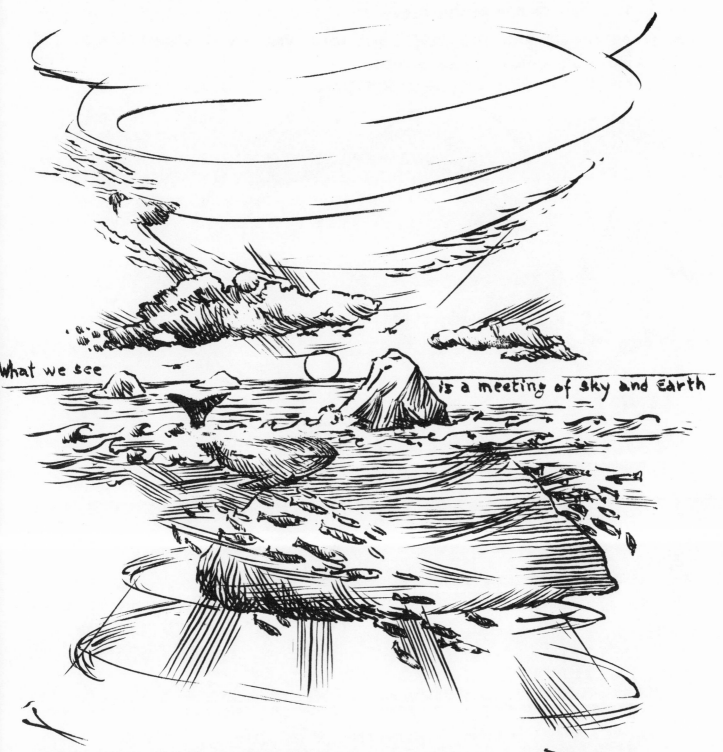 is a meeting of sky and Earth

Not visible to the eye are the infinite uncreated abilities
of the under- and over-worlds. We are able to see a little bit up
and a little bit down into these spheres by diving down or flying up.
We know the waves of oceans and how they are born out of their
depths and how the main body of the iceberg is hidden to the eye.
What we do and say is only a slither of what we think and only
a millimeter of the miles to come out of the womb of time...

The Void Scape of the face
earring's Angels pull your skull down and your inner space lifts
as if blown by wind. Look down ...

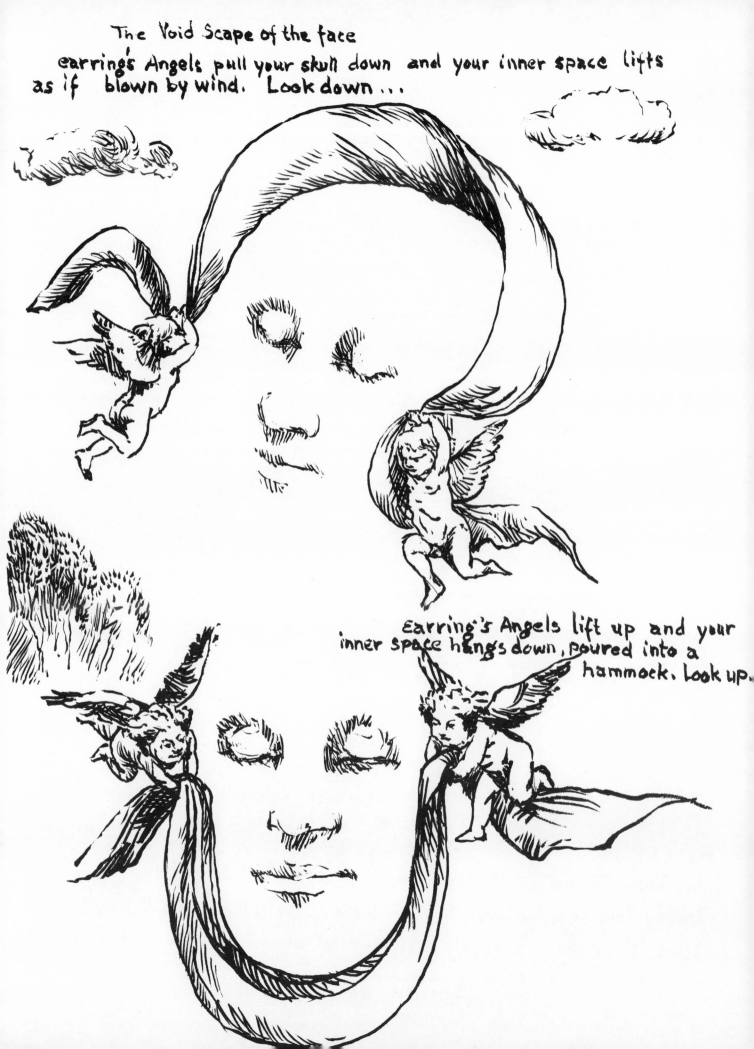

Earring's Angels lift up and your
inner space hangs down, poured into a
hammock. Look up.

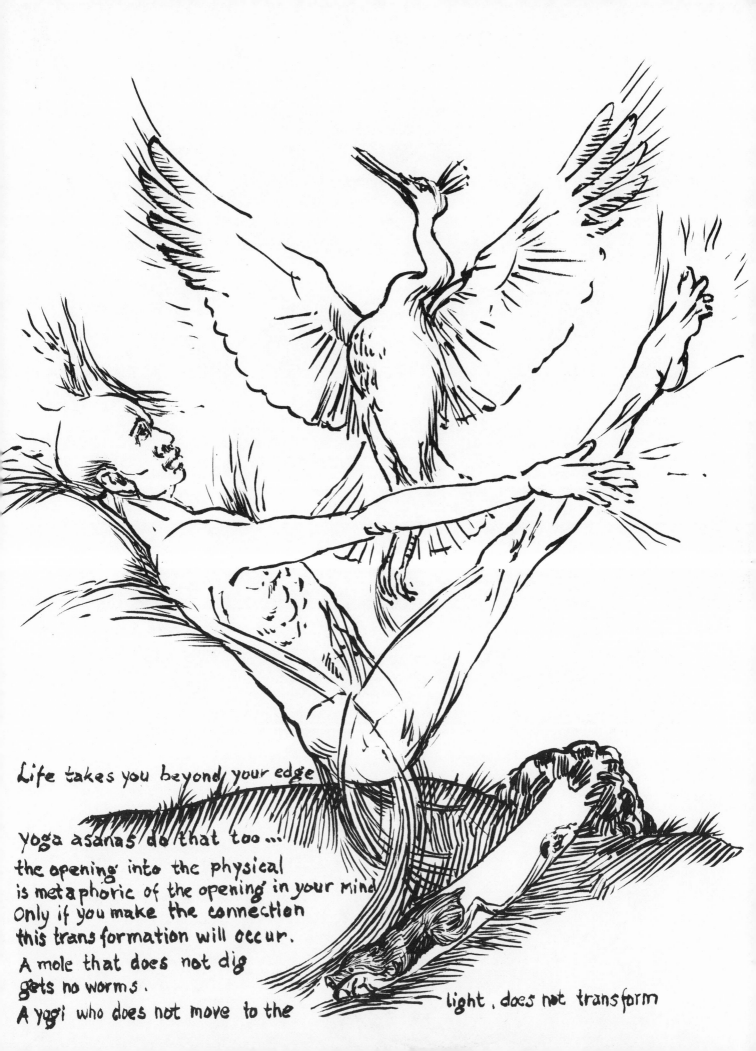

Life takes you beyond your edge

Yoga asanas do that too...
the opening into the physical
is metaphoric of the opening in your mind
Only if you make the connection
this transformation will occur.
A mole that does not dig
gets no worms.
A yogi who does not move to the   light, does not transform

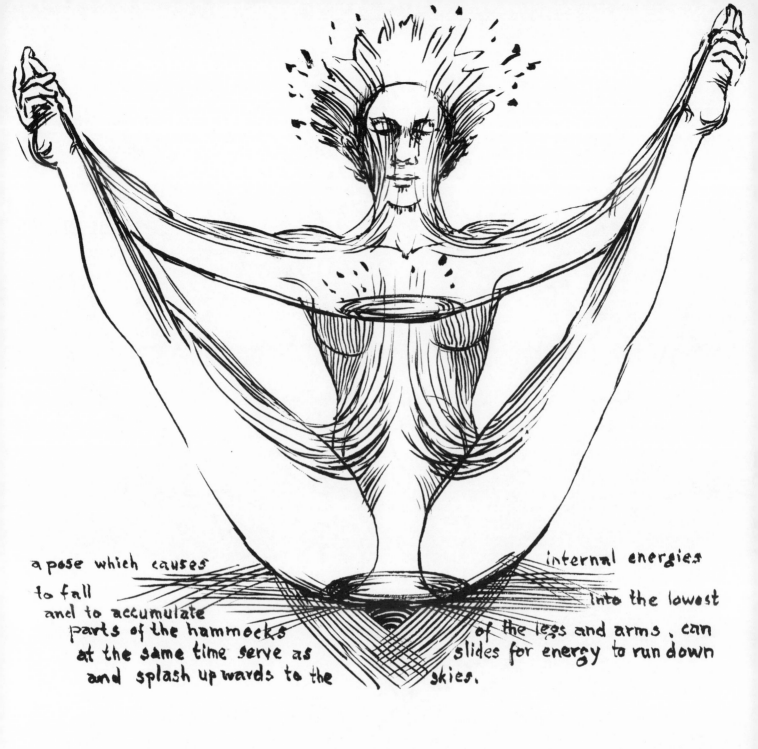

a pose which causes
to fall
and to accumulate
parts of the hammocks
at the same time serve as
and splash upwards to the

internal energies
into the lowest
of the legs and arms, can
slides for energy to run down
skies.

The jelly fish is the
doughnut of the ocean.
Contained water in
motion;
a brain floating in
meditation.

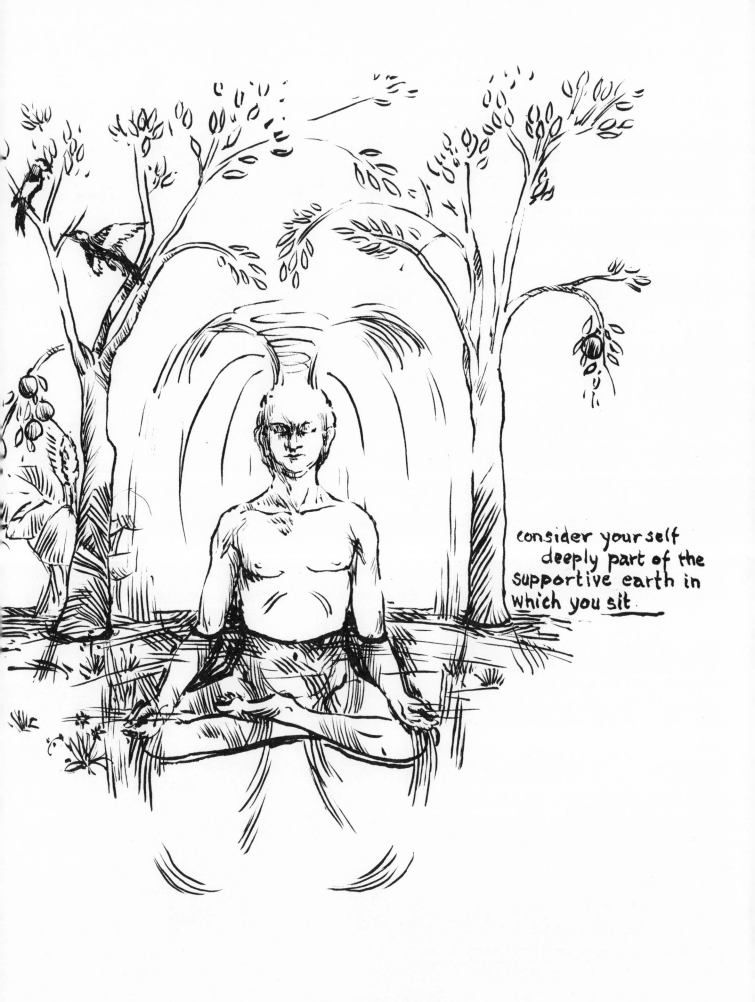

consider yourself
deeply part of the
supportive earth in
which you sit

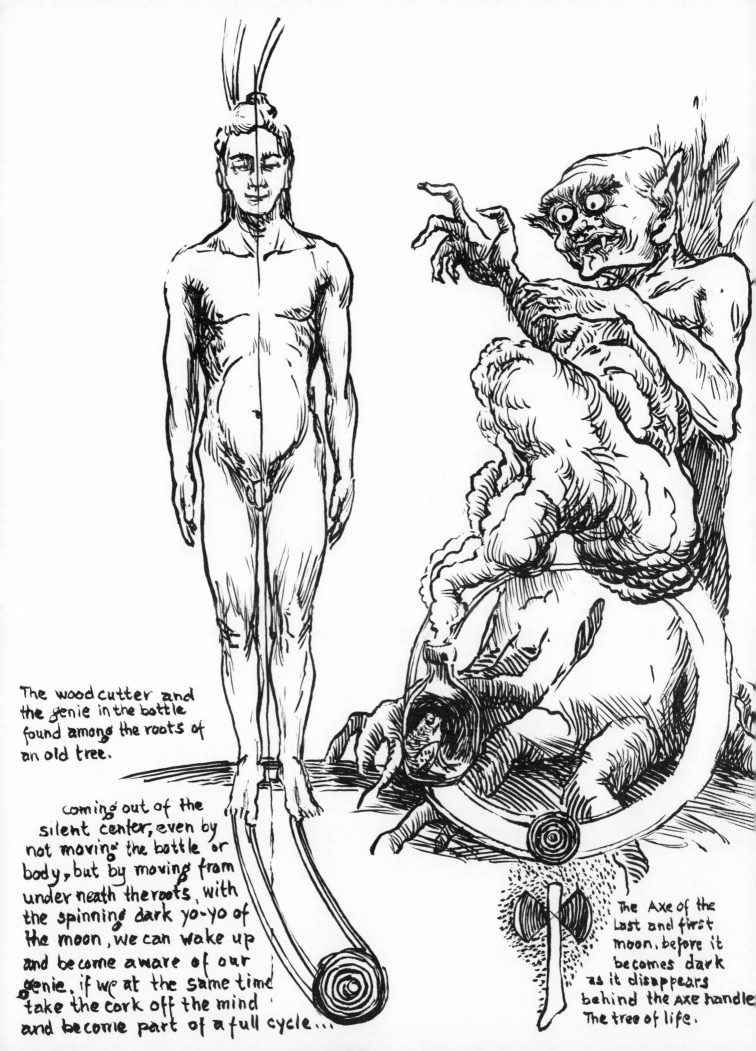

The wood cutter and
the genie in the bottle
found among the roots of
an old tree.

coming out of the
silent center, even by
not moving the bottle or
body, but by moving from
under neath the roots, with
the spinning dark yo-yo of
the moon, we can wake up
and become aware of our
genie, if we at the same time
take the cork off the mind
and become part of a full cycle...

The Axe of the
Last and first
moon, before it
becomes dark
as it disappears
behind the axe handle
The tree of life.

Hold on to nothing.

When our soul gets caught and put into an other form that does not fit, the restrictions will cause unhappiness. Our physical health gets broken down. No doctor will be able to cure it, until we learn to trust our own body's wisdom. The body was built by the soul. It has all it needs to maintain itself, as long as it stays in contact with its maker. Move the body with a listening mind.
Be in Yoga.

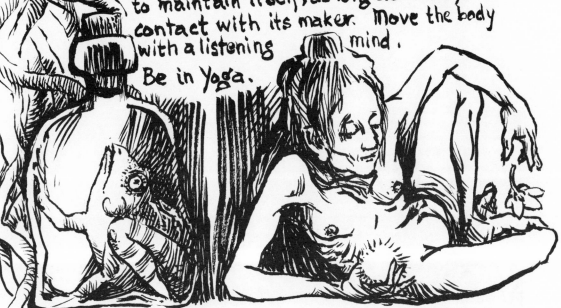

free from all restrictions does not mean that there are no restrictions... Just not holding on to anything.

hidden, overgrown by roots he found a small glass bottle with a cork in the opening. let me out!, a tiny voice begged.

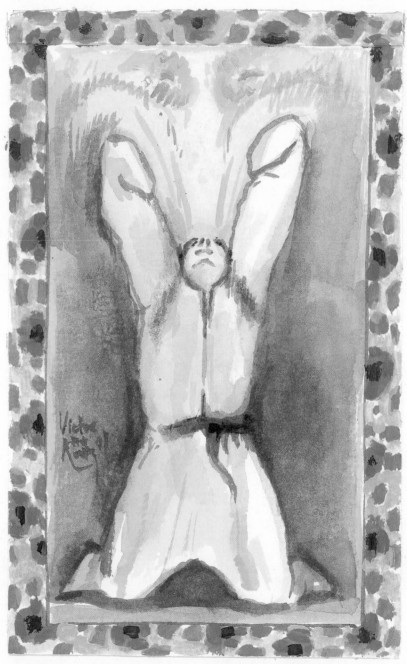

opening up to a power placed higher...

one-direction mind
versus
A Panoramic view

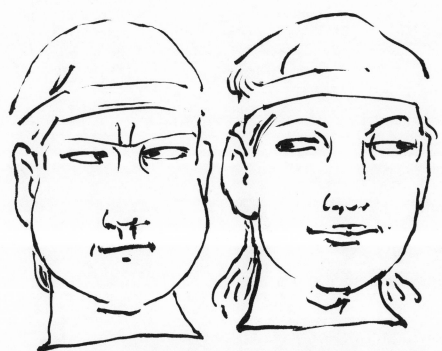

a focused   mind - the masculine - yang: forever into the same
direction, penetrating deeper and deeper into matter
one point - all of the time.

It is just a matter of stepping back, let space in and see
where you are, what you are ...

Ariadne's thread — the yogic connection.
The panoramic view that gives us a   chance to scan
the situation and allows us to move   freely into
whatever direction, without getting   lost in the
labyrinth of the Body-Mind-World.

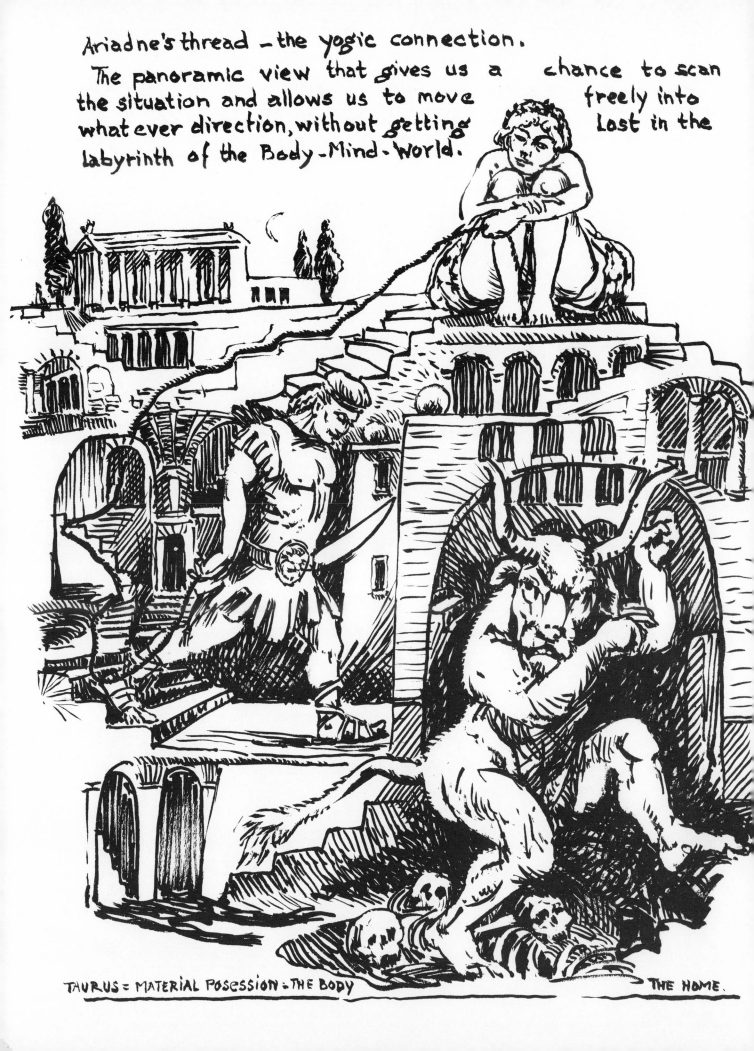

TAURUS = MATERIAL POSESSION = THE BODY   THE HOME.

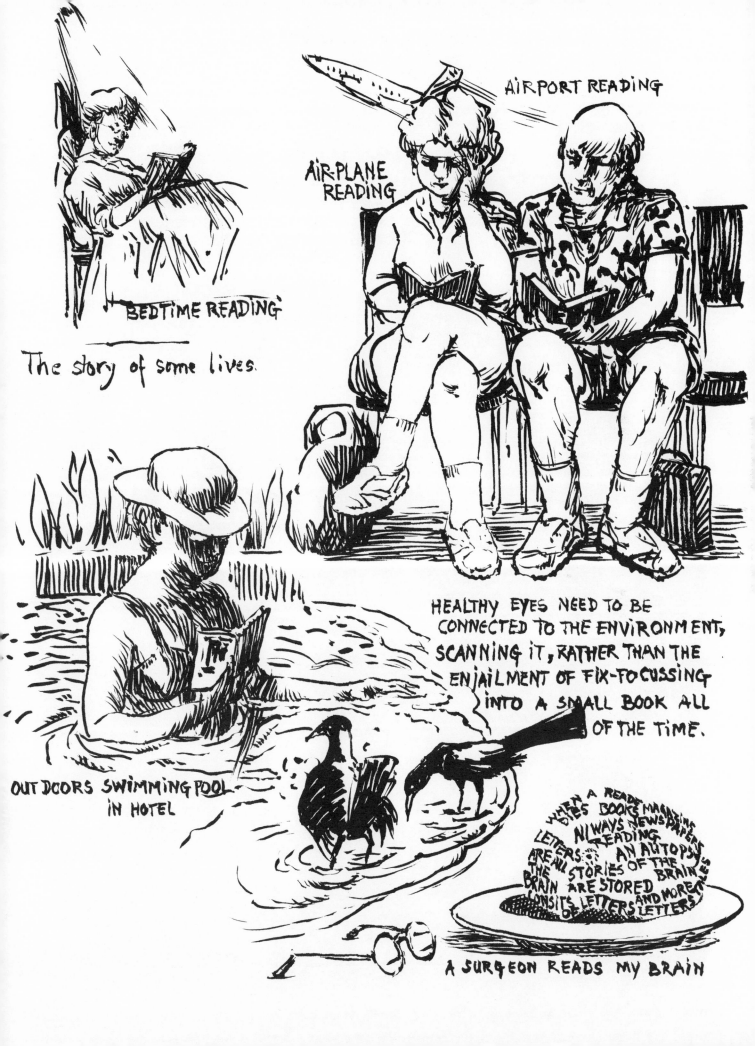

BEDTIME READING

The story of some lives.

AIRPLANE READING

AIRPORT READING

OUTDOORS SWIMMING POOL IN HOTEL

HEALTHY EYES NEED TO BE CONNECTED TO THE ENVIRONMENT, SCANNING IT, RATHER THAN THE ENJAILMENT OF FIX-FOCUSSING INTO A SMALL BOOK ALL OF THE TIME.

WHEN A READER DIES BOOKS MAGAZINES ALWAYS NEWSPAPERS READING LETTERS AN AUTOPSY ARE ALL STORIES OF THE THE BRAIN BRAIN ARE STORED AND MORE TALES CONSISTS OF LETTERS LETTERS

A SURGEON READS MY BRAIN

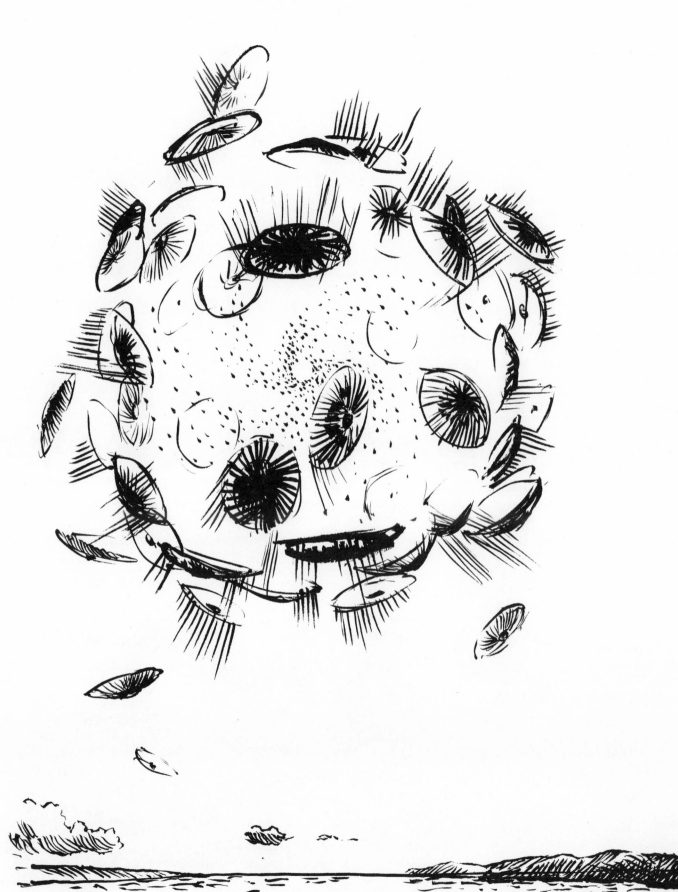

When seeing falls away, the eye sees its inner light.

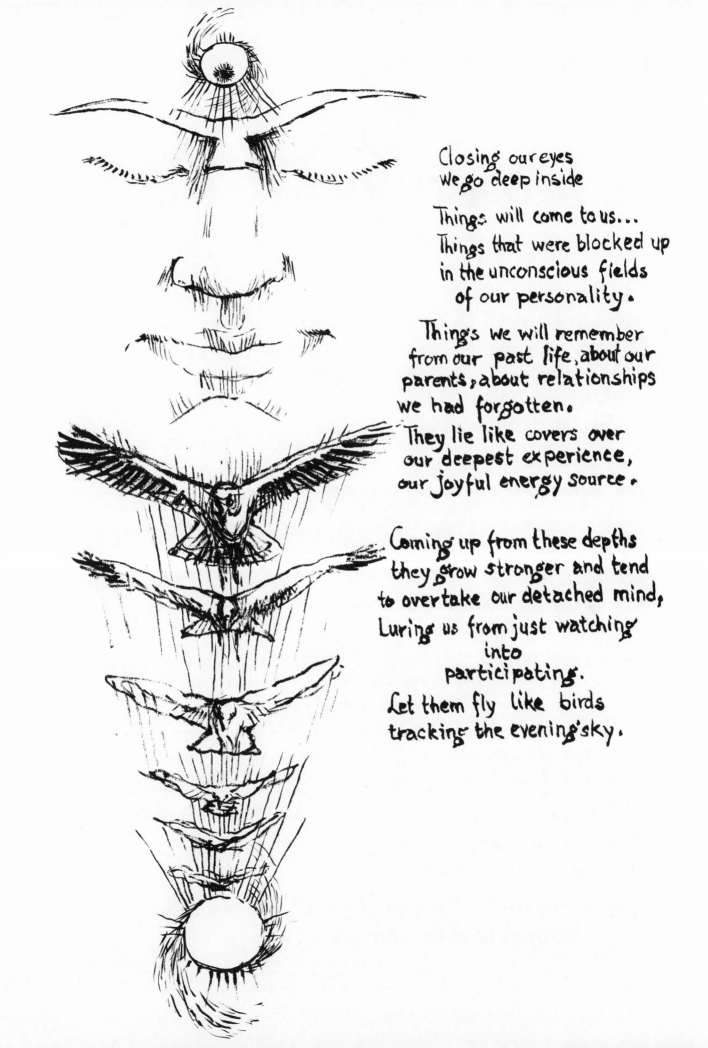

Closing our eyes
we go deep inside

Things will come to us...
Things that were blocked up
in the unconscious fields
of our personality.

Things we will remember
from our past life, about our
parents, about relationships
we had forgotten.
They lie like covers over
our deepest experience,
our joyful energy source.

Coming up from these depths
they grow stronger and tend
to overtake our detached mind,
Luring us from just watching
into
participating.
Let them fly like birds
tracking the evening sky.

Ode to John Lennon.

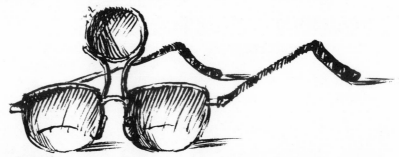

Third-eye glasses are not going to be of any help.

No implants of silicone, of hair, of hearing aids,
No Yoga exercises. No Saints. No Concert tickets.
No books, No Bible, No Bhagavad Gita.
    Anything you pick up
    Anything you want to have
                in order to be ...
There is No way to behave.
You already have what you sincerely are deep inside
            You belong to your creator
            All you have to do, is accept.

Listen inside
See inside
for nothing out there can help you
if you don't help yourself to accept what you are
                and have always been,
            the original you
            can't be repeated
No techniques. No science can help you.
Third-eye glasses are not going to be of any help
    and if John is shyly including Yoko in the end,
he tells you that you too can find and accept your Soul mate.
Everything changes. Nothing can be repeated.
Nothing stays the same.

Your acceptance is not going to last forever either,
        unless it becomes your lifestyle.

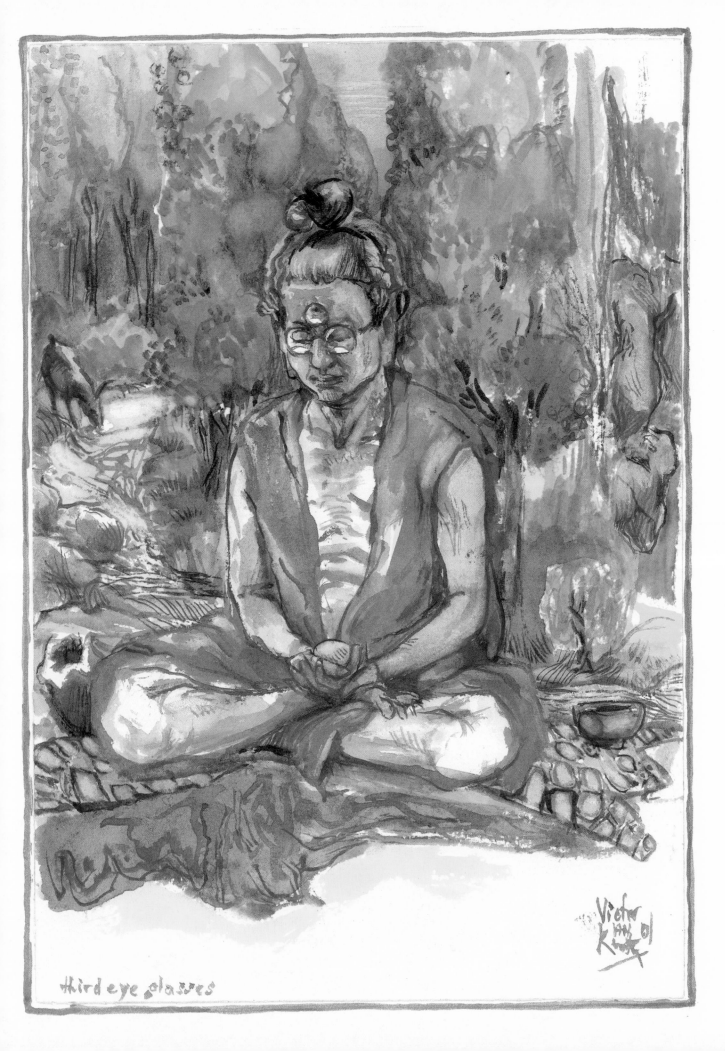

third eye glasses

disconnected, it becomes schizophrenic,
    connected, it becomes the Truth.

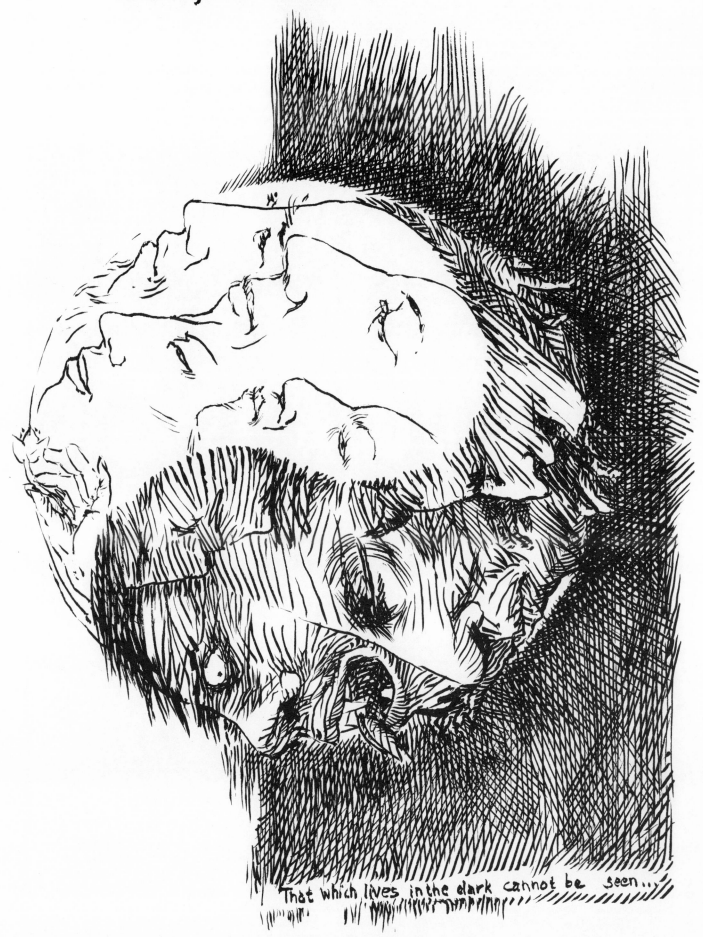

That which lives in the dark cannot be seen...
    Truth.

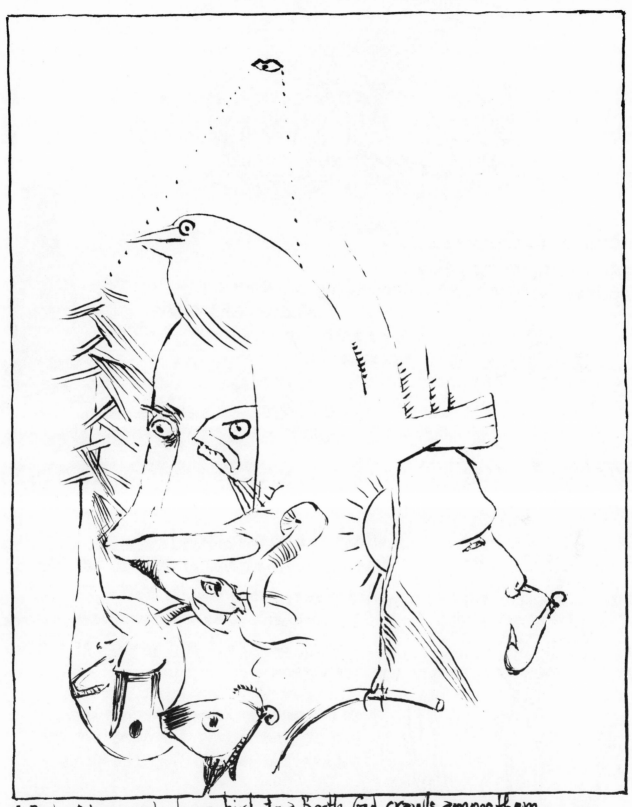

to Birds, God can only be a bird, to a Beetle God crawls among them
the God of Flowers has many coloured petals, to Fishes God swims and calls
you back with his bait. According to man God made him after his own
Image. If we only knew who we really are besides Ignorance...

Limited by the outer eye

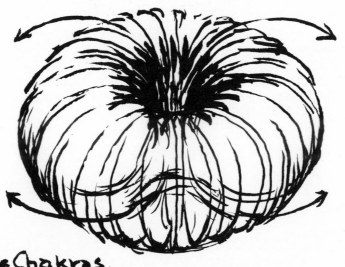

The masculine Chakras.
   activating energy flow
   either up- or down, depending on where you unfold:
                    above or below
             spreading your bundle, out of
             your basket

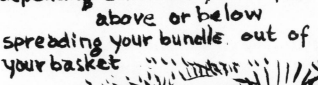

Watch the human body form.
Our streaming energy shaped us like a
wild river, changing its bed.
   It happens when we are very active,
during our restless youth, or pumping
iron, etc.
   Wherever the body narrows,
at the ankles, knees, perineum,
waist and neck, is where we can
locate the masculine chakras.

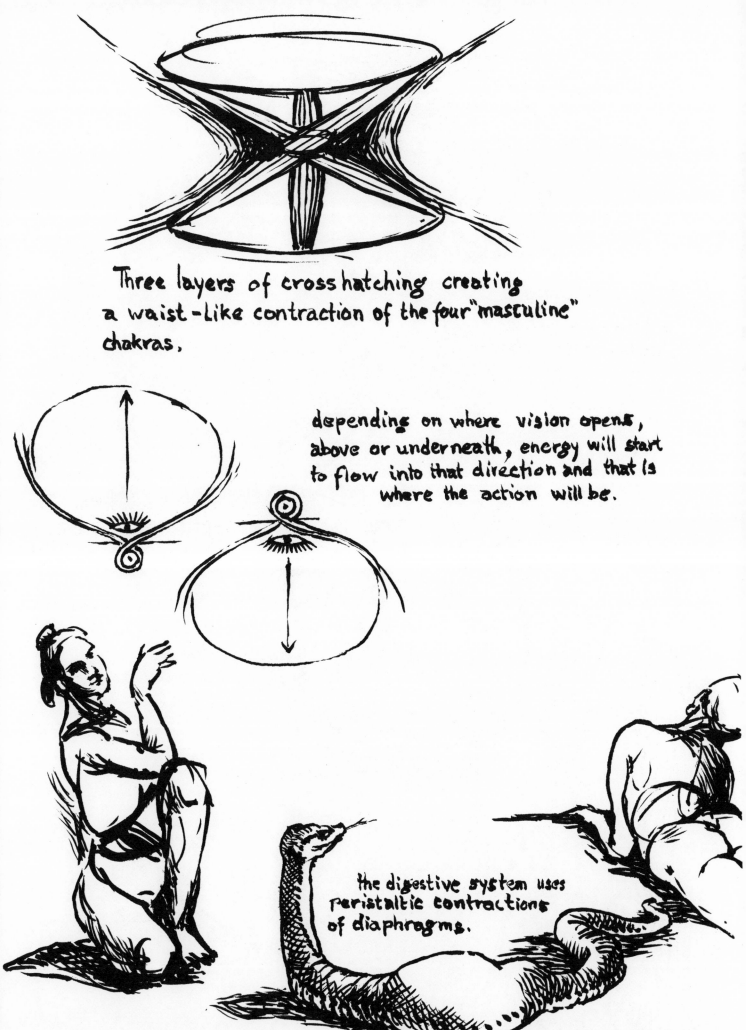

Three layers of cross hatching creating
a waist-like contraction of the four "masculine"
chakras,

depending on where vision opens,
above or underneath, energy will start
to flow into that direction and that is
where the action will be.

the digestive system uses
peristaltic contractions
of diaphragms.

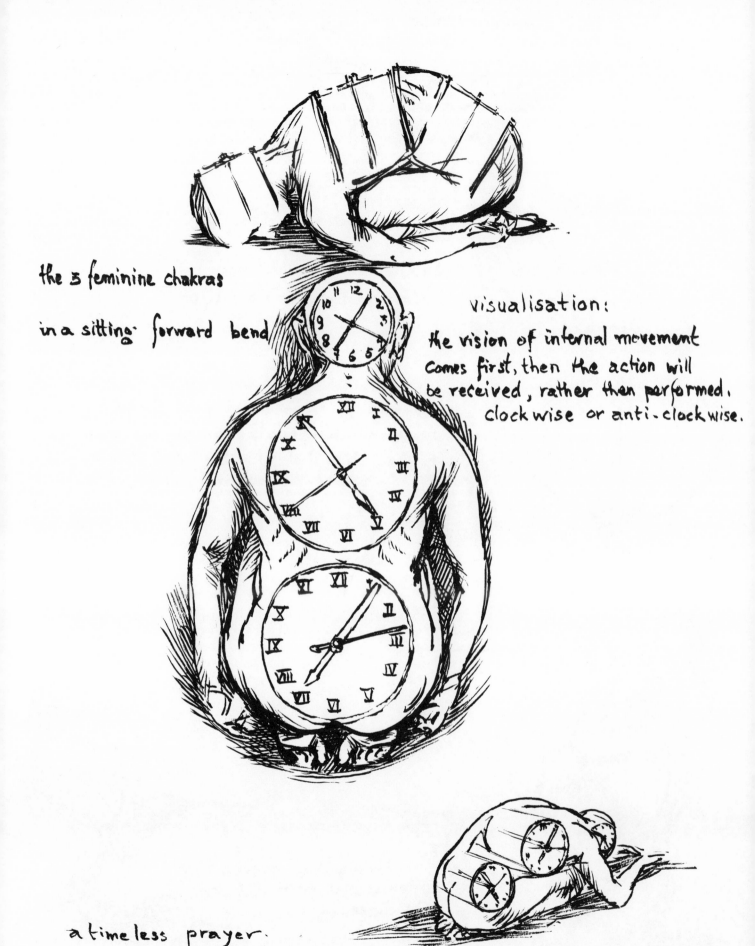

the 3 feminine chakras

in a sitting forward bend

visualisation:

the vision of internal movement
comes first, then the action will
be received, rather then performed.
clockwise or anti-clockwise.

a timeless prayer.

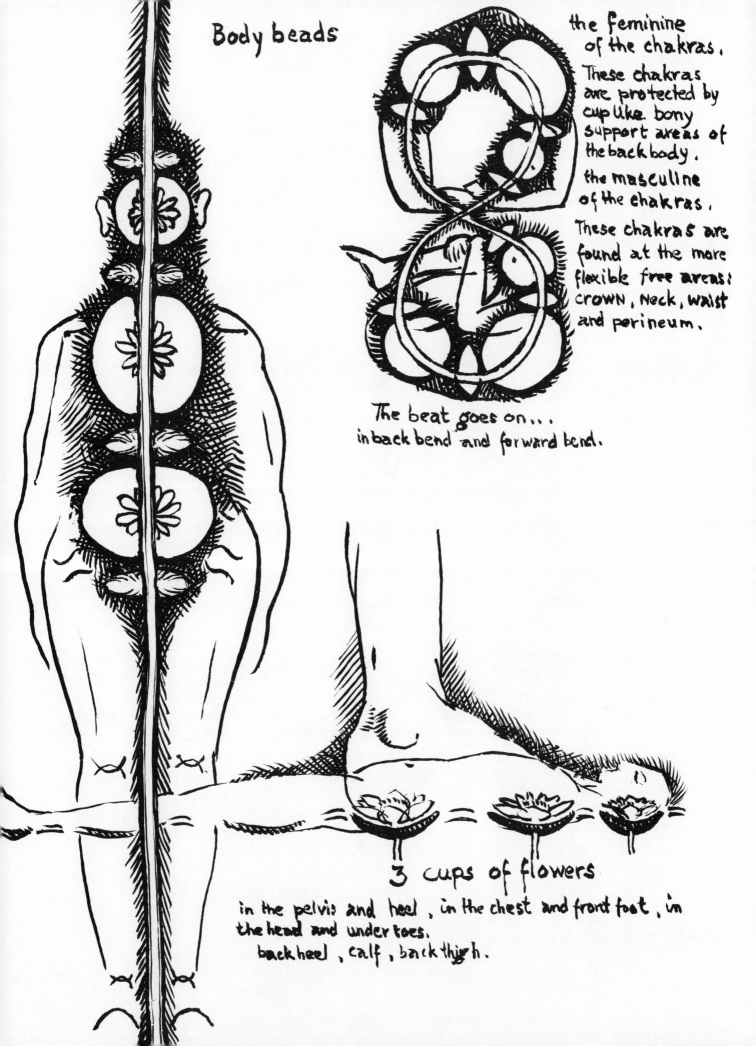

Body beads

the feminine of the chakras. These chakras are protected by cup like bony support areas of the back body.

the masculine of the chakras.

These chakras are found at the more flexible free areas: crown, neck, waist and perineum.

The beat goes on... in back bend and forward bend.

3 cups of flowers

in the pelvis and heel, in the chest and front foot, in the head and under toes.

back heel, calf, back thigh.

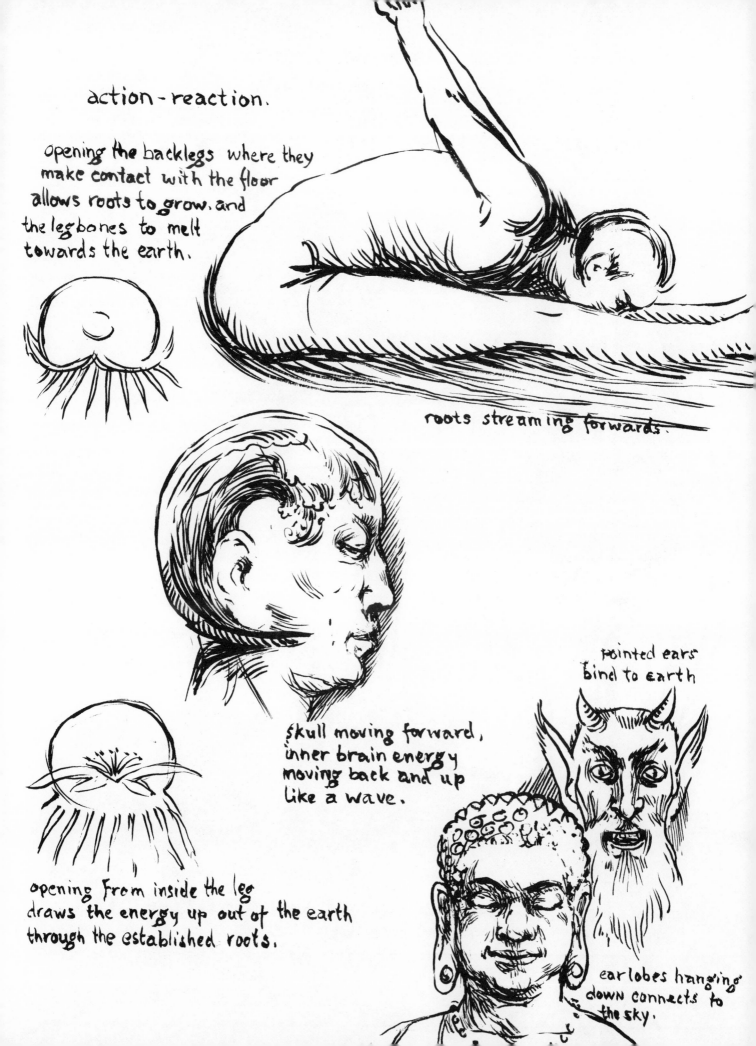

action-reaction.

opening the backlegs where they
make contact with the floor
allows roots to grow. and
the legbones to melt
towards the earth.

roots streaming forwards.

skull moving forward,
inner brain energy
moving back and up
like a wave.

opening from inside the leg
draws the energy up out of the earth
through the established roots.

pointed ears
bind to earth

earlobes hanging
down connects to
the sky.

growing an elephant's trunk
by unwinding the brain of the
body mind while observing the
breath.

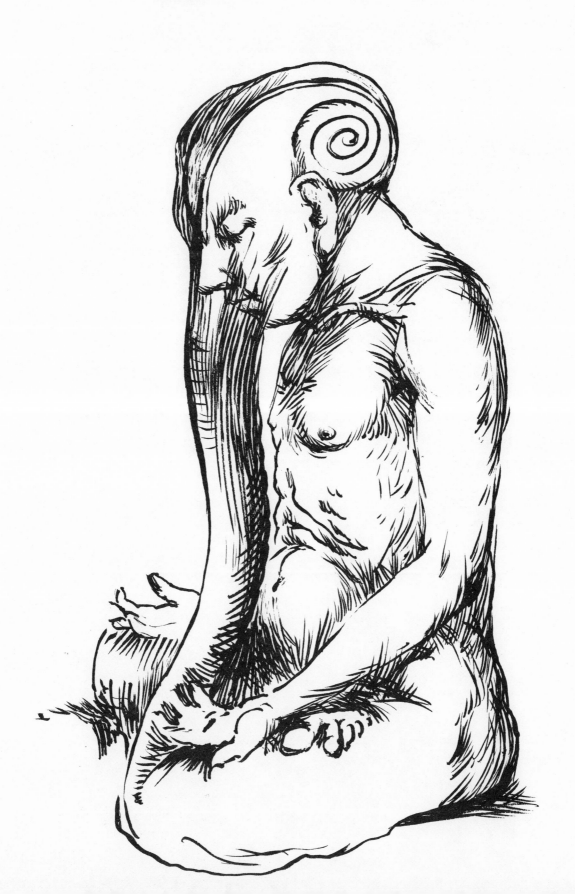

EVERYTHING HAPPENS AT ONCE.
To be able to witness this, we have
to find and be in our silent center.

SKY

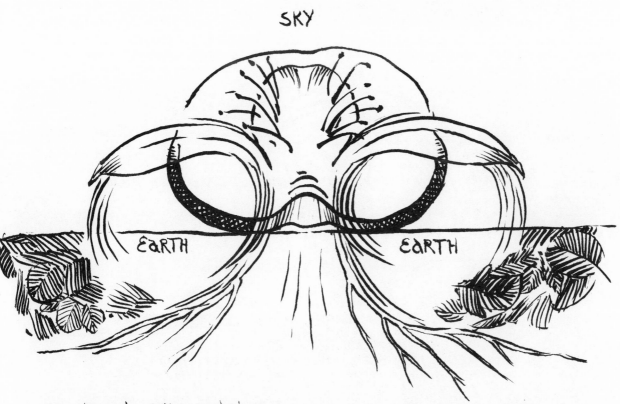

EARTH   EARTH

the Bowl of the pelvis
has to root down into the earth, to bring up the energy into
and through the sacrum and open the chakra-flower out
and down, its petals folding to nourish back into the earth.

Out of dust we are born,
Back to dust we will return.

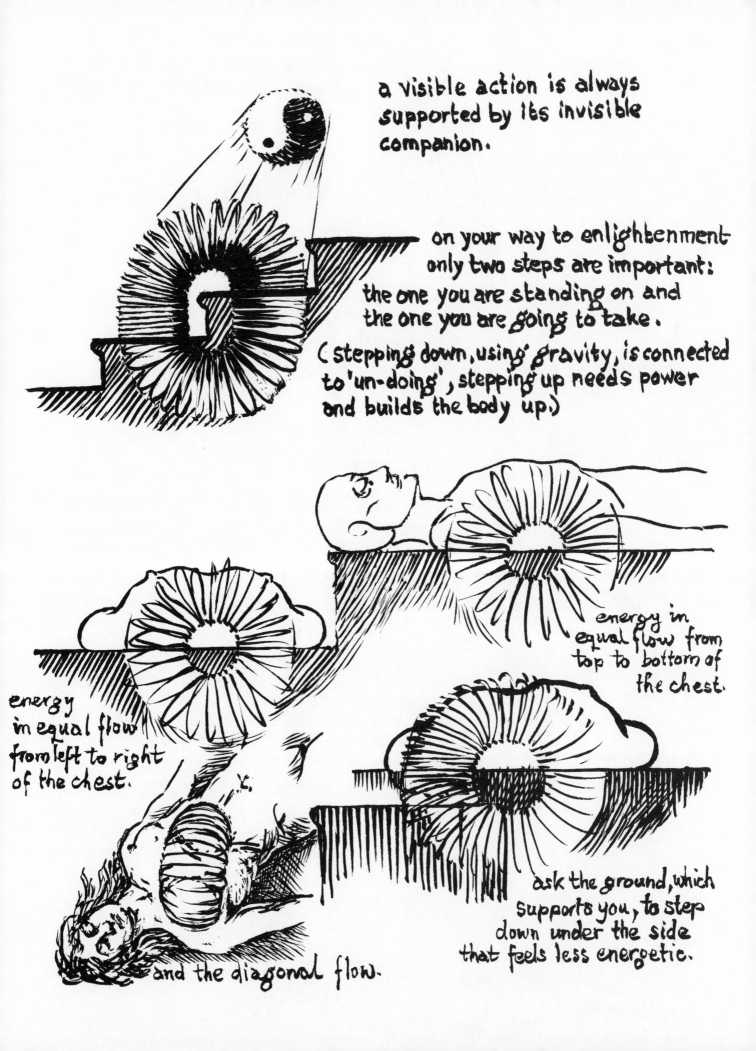

a visible action is always
supported by its invisible
companion.

on your way to enlightenment
only two steps are important:
the one you are standing on and
the one you are going to take.

(stepping down, using gravity, is connected
to 'un-doing', stepping up needs power
and builds the body up.)

energy in
equal flow from
top to bottom of
the chest.

energy
in equal flow
from left to right
of the chest.

ask the ground, which
supports you, to step
down under the side
that feels less energetic.

and the diagonal flow.

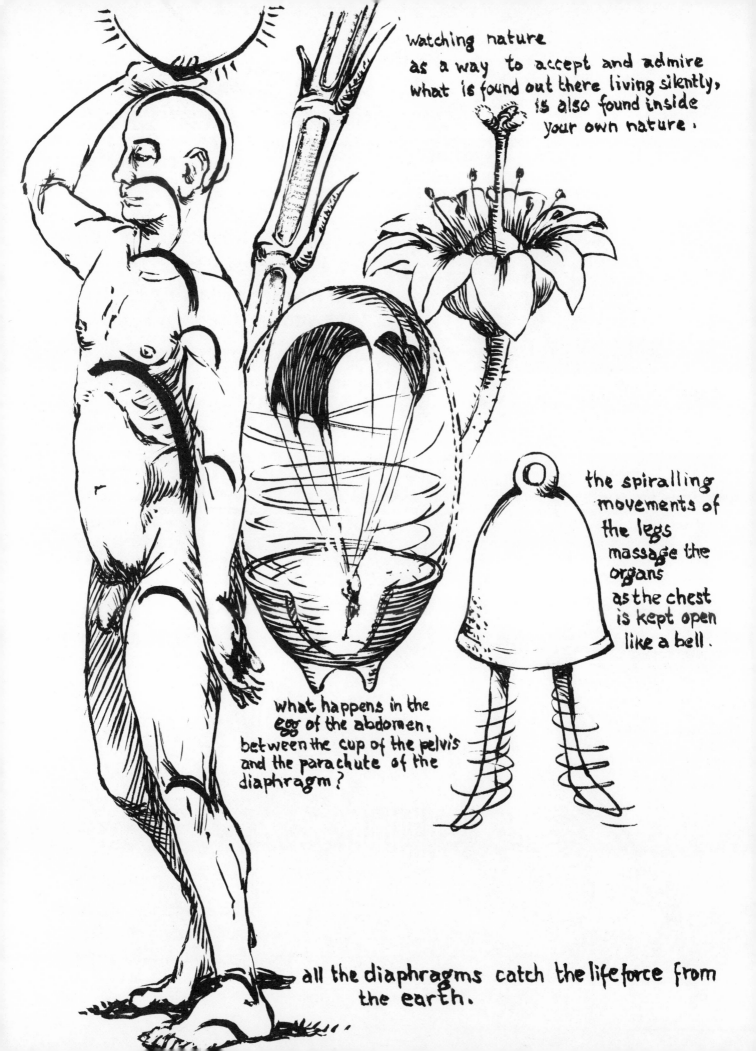

watching nature
as a way to accept and admire
what is found out there living silently,
is also found inside
your own nature.

the spiralling
movements of
the legs
massage the
organs
as the chest
is kept open
like a bell.

what happens in the
egg of the abdomen,
between the cup of the pelvis
and the parachute of the
diaphragm?

all the diaphragms catch the life force from
the earth.

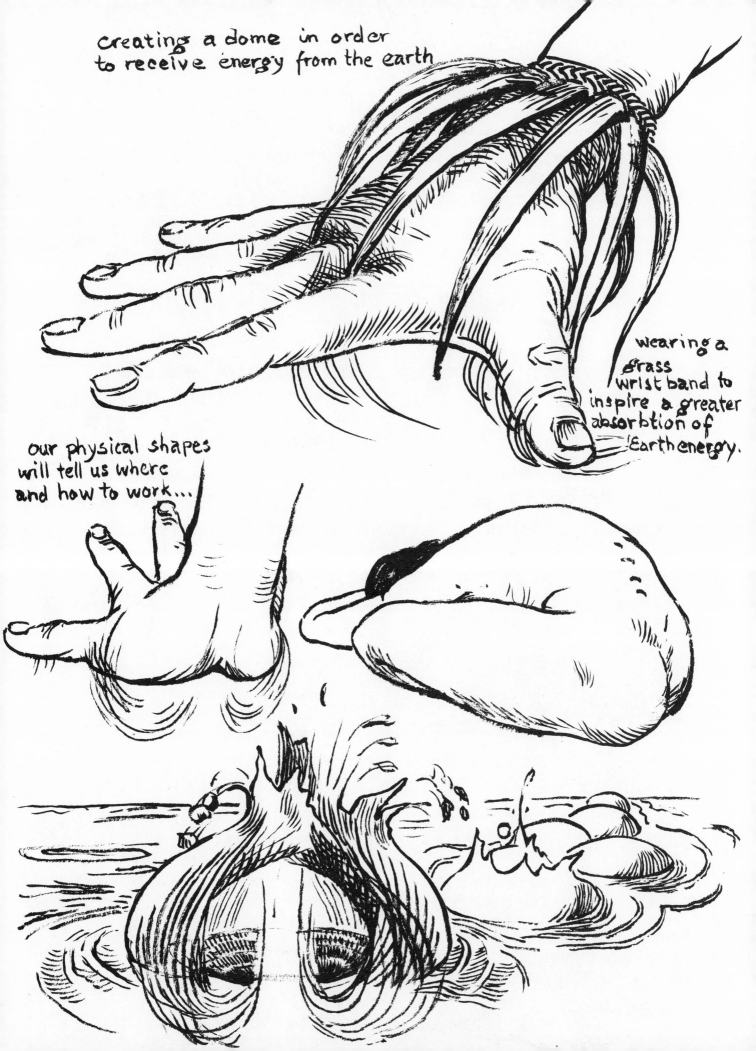

creating a dome in order
to receive energy from the earth

wearing a
grass
wrist band to
inspire a greater
absorbtion of
Earth energy.

our physical shapes
will tell us where
and how to work...

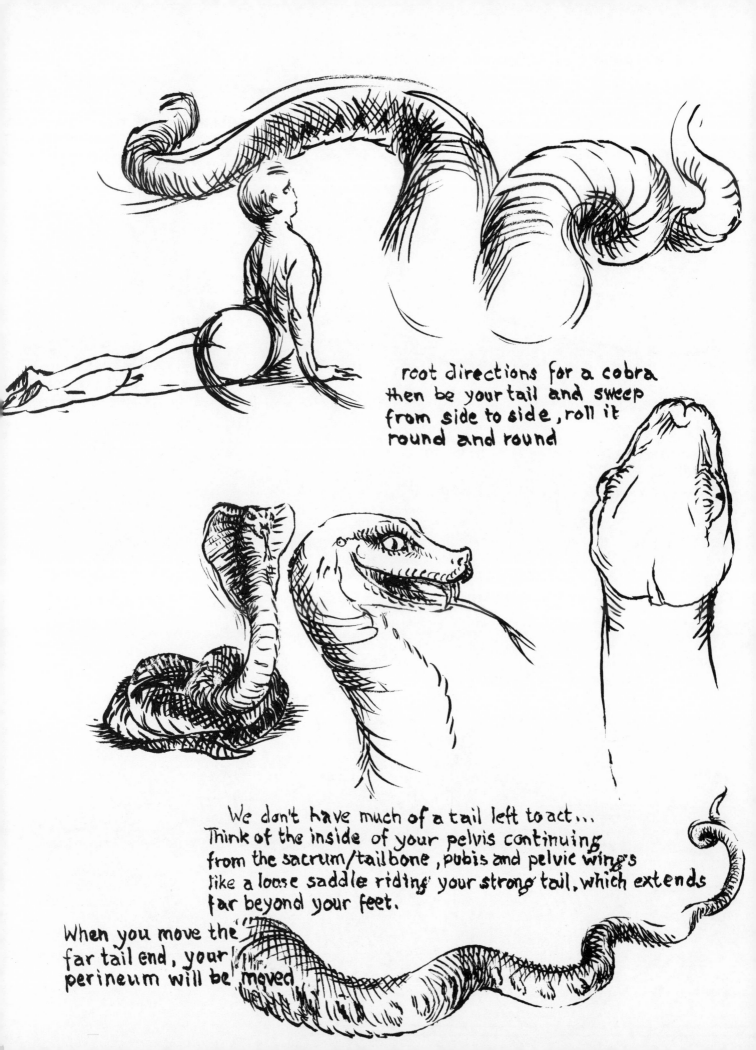

root directions for a cobra
then be your tail and sweep
from side to side, roll it
round and round

We don't have much of a tail left to act...
Think of the inside of your pelvis continuing
from the sacrum/tailbone, pubis and pelvic wings
like a loose saddle riding your strong tail, which extends
far beyond your feet.

When you move the
far tail end, your
perineum will be moved

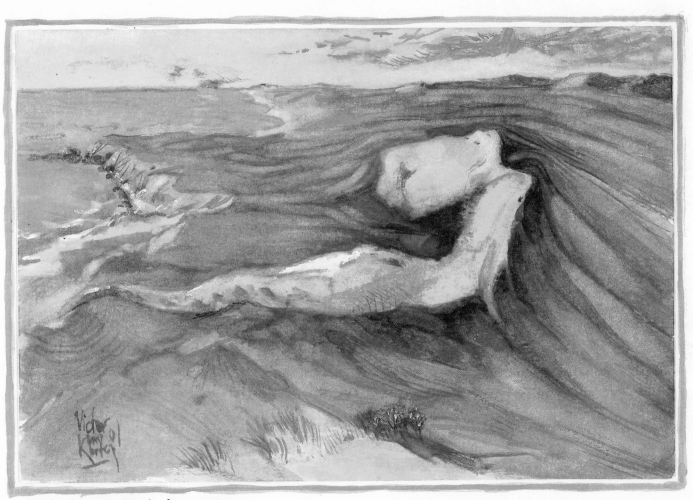

reach through the bodyscape.

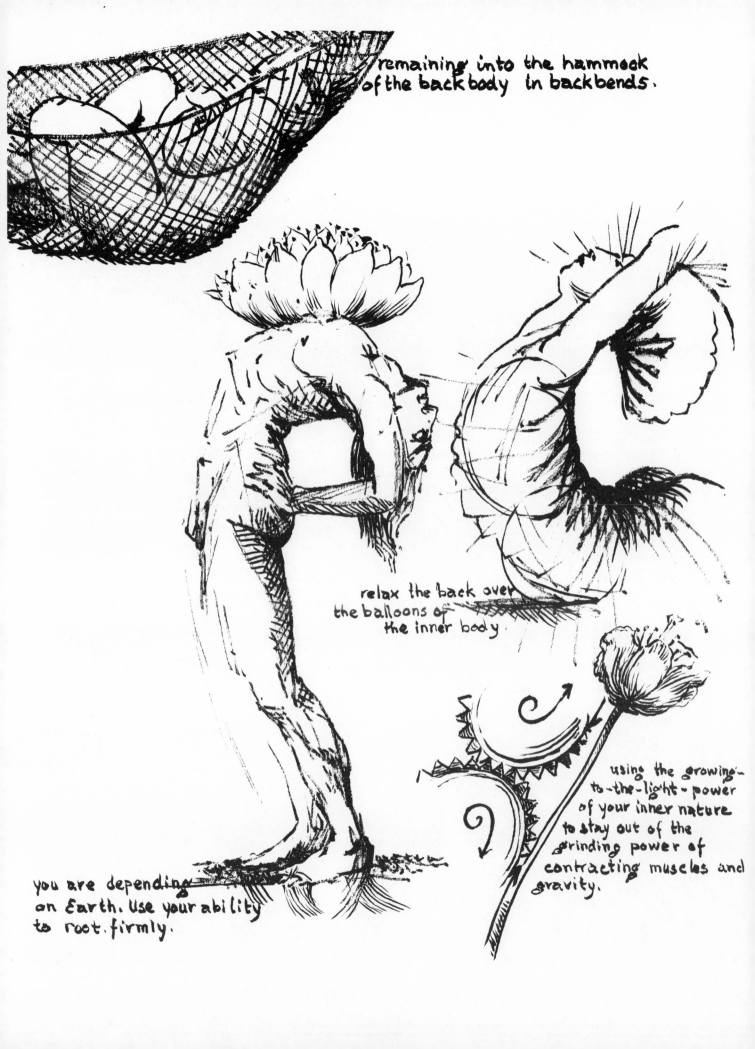

remaining into the hammock
of the back body in backbends.

relax the back over
the balloons of
the inner body

using the growing-
to-the-light-power
of your inner nature
to stay out of the
grinding power of
contracting muscles and
gravity.

you are depending
on Earth. Use your ability
to root firmly.

the Crawling Spine
in action.

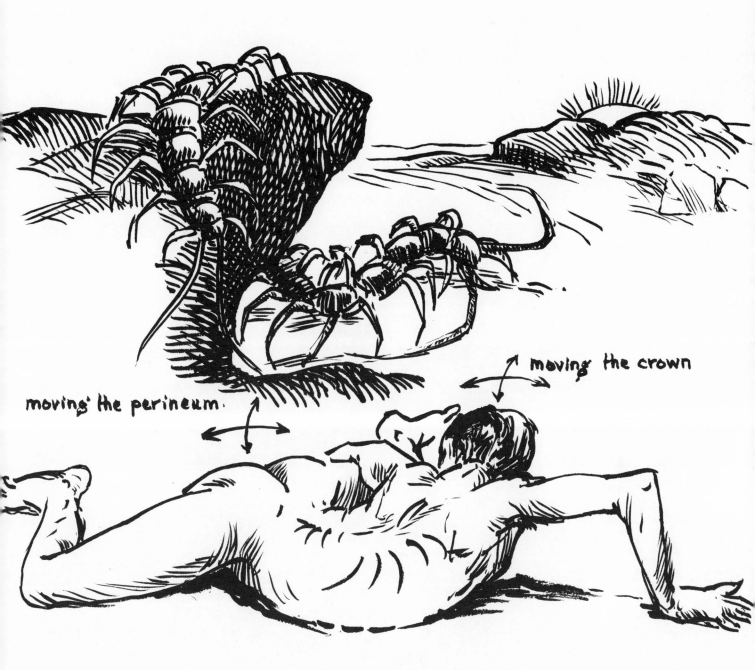

moving the crown

moving the perineum.

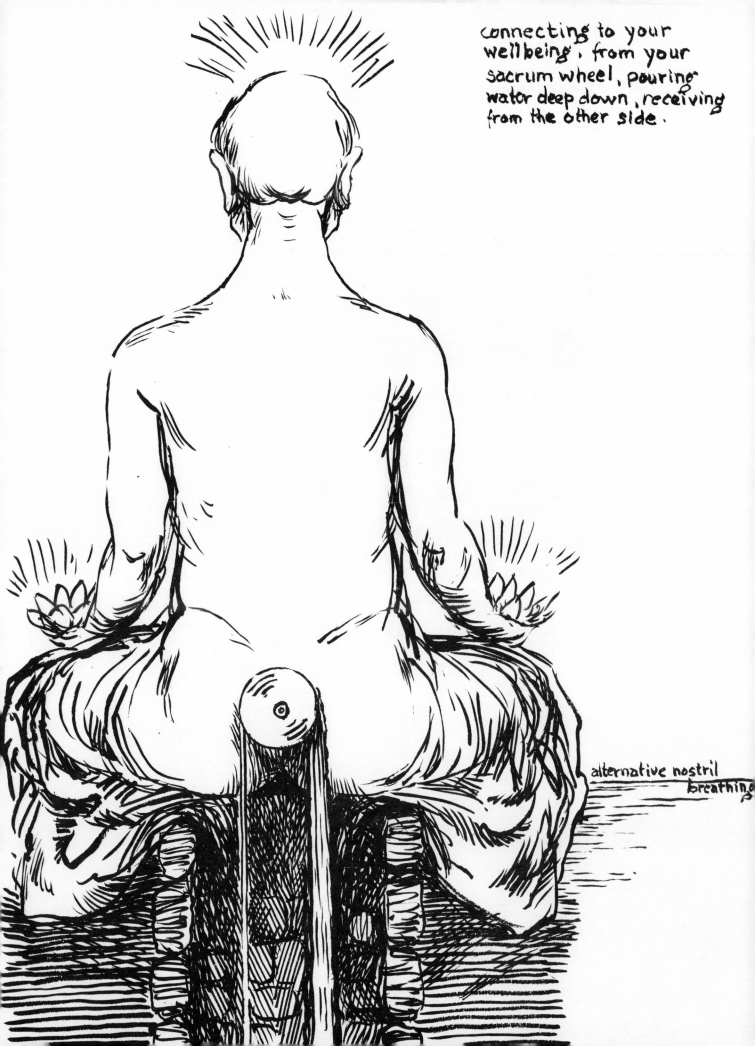

connecting to your wellbeing, from your sacrum wheel, pouring water deep down, receiving from the other side.

alternative nostril breathing

using the vision of the living space of the pelvis
to settle into a comfortable sitting pose
watching the breath coming into different parts of the inner body
and the nostrils by allowing the energy to pour into diffent areas
of the earth, making the wheel spin in different directions.

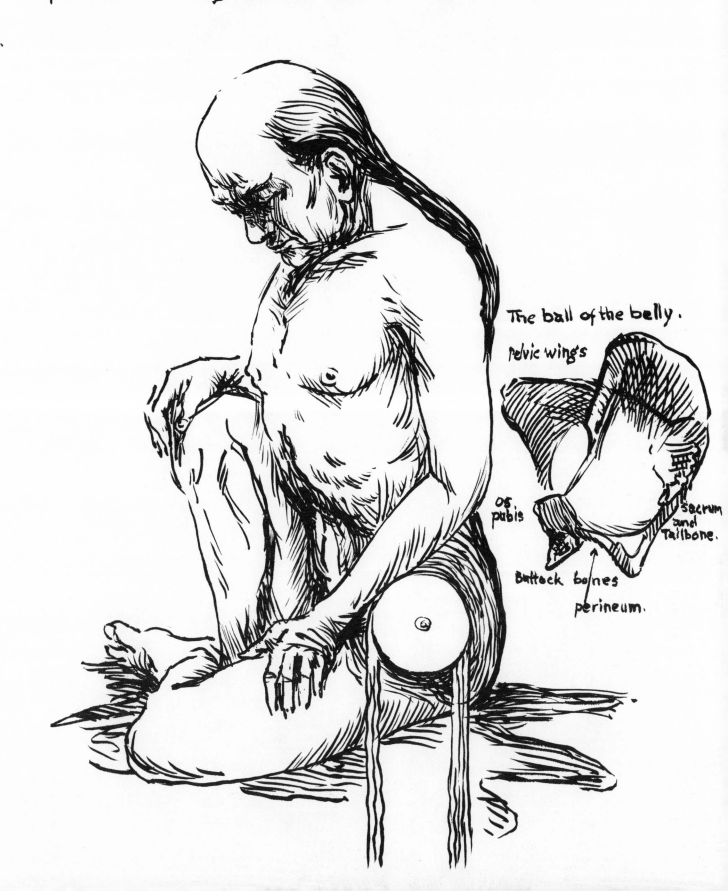

The ball of the belly.

pelvic wings

os pubis

sacrum and Tailbone.

Buttock bones

perineum.

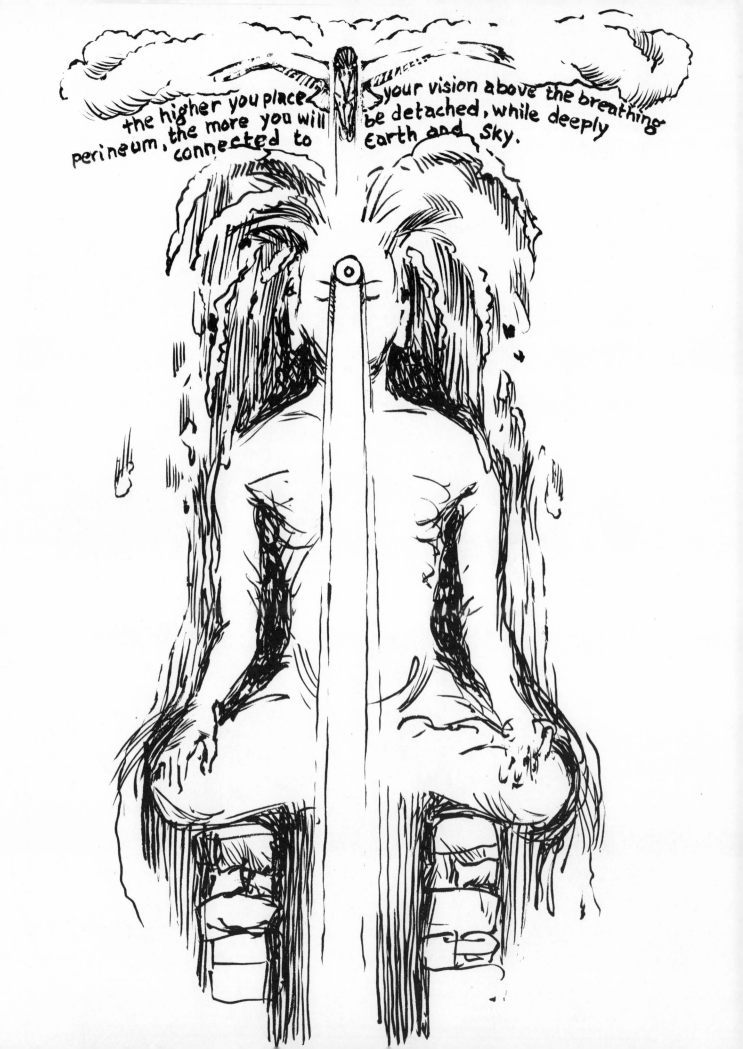

the higher you place your vision above the breathing perineum, the more you will be detached, while deeply connected to Earth and Sky.